Reason and Passion

Reason and Passion

*A Celebration of
the Work of
Hanna Segal*

David Bell
Editor

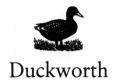

Duckworth

First published in 1997 by
Gerald Duckworth & Co. Ltd.
The Old Piano Factory
48 Hoxton Square, London N1 6PB
Tel: 0171 729 5986
Fax: 0171 729 0015

A catalogue record for this book is available
from the British Library.

ISBN 0 7156 2803 8

Typeset by Ray Davies
Printed in Great Britain by
Redwood Books Ltd, Trowbridge

Contents

Preface

Since it was founded in 1920, the Tavistock Clinic has developed a wide range of psychotherapeutic approaches to community mental health which have always been strongly influenced by psychoanalysis. In the last thirty years it has also developed systemic family therapy as a new theoretical model and clinical approach to family problems. The Clinic has become the largest training institution in Britain for work of this kind, providing post-graduate and qualifying courses in social work, psychology, psychiatry, child, adolescent and adult psychotherapy and, latterly, in nursing. It trains about 1,200 students each year in over 45 courses.

The Clinic's philosophy has been one of influencing mental health work toward therapeutic and humane methods and has, as an aim, the dissemination of training, clinical expertise and research throughout Britain and the rest of the world. This major new series will make available the clinical and theoretical work that has been most influential at the Tavistock Clinic. It will also present new approaches in the understanding and treatment of psychological disturbance in children, adolescents and adults, as individuals and in families.

Reason and Passion is a collection of papers by a group of leading psychoanalysts who have been inspired by the work of Hanna Segal. Set in the context of a biographical introduction by the editor, each paper makes a personal contribution to furthering the theoretical and clinical ideas in her thinking. These ideas have been widely influential in the work of the Tavistock Clinic and thereby in the whole field of mental health.

Nicholas Temple and Margot Waddell
Series Editors

Man is but a reed ... but he is a thinking reed
                              Blaise Pascal (1623-1662)

I have striven not to laugh at human actions, not to weep at them nor
to hate them, but to understand them
                              Baruch Spinoza (1663-1677)

Foreword

Hanna Segal needs no introduction. From the time that she qualified as an analyst in 1946 and four years later at the age of thirty-one as a Training Analyst, she has been outstandingly distinguished as an original thinker and contributor. This is reflected in her much appreciated articles and books and in her contributions as a gifted analyst and teacher within our Society and in many other parts of the world. She was President of our Society in 1977, the year in which she was also Freud Professor at University College, London. She was again acting-President of the Society in 1981, and twice Vice-President of the International Psychoanalytical Association. In 1994 she was awarded the Sigourney Weaver prize for her outstanding contribution to psychoanalysis. She is one of the most distinguished living psychoanalysts and the finest exponent of the work of Melanie Klein.

Hanna Segal brings to psychoanalytic work an incisive clarity of mind, together with a deep human understanding and a very special capacity to cut through the superficial to what really matters. David Bell's extensive introduction to this book provides an account of her contributions to psychoanalytic theory and practice and gives a picture of her as a person. The high level of her scientific achievement is unquestioned even by those who may not always agree with her.

I am particularly delighted with the title of the book, *Reason and Passion*, since Hanna Segal is notably able to combine these qualities herself. She is fiercely loyal to those people and ideas she cares about: I remember her joking – 'I react like a tiger when my loved ones are under attack'. Yet that would be to understate her strength and real capacity to bear and work through problems and take on the task, emotionally and intellectually, of looking after and developing what she believes in. This has always been so much the case that many of us have come to rely on her to hear and think through problems and difficult issues. She has been a great midwife to the creative contributions of others.

She is full blooded both in her approach to life and in her approach to psychoanalysis. Her great zest for life comes over in her teaching, as in her written work and in her way of living. She is as intensely engaged in her professional life as in her family and personal life. In the British Psycho-Analytical Society, she is not only greatly respected, but also much loved. She has always been available to be turned to for a thoughtful and valued opinion in difficult times. So it was especially appropriate that in 1996 our members welcomed her as an honorary, or rather Honoured Member of our Society, as it is now timely that a book dedicated to her, develops her contributions to psychoanalysis.

I feel especially privileged, personally and on behalf of the British Psycho-Analytical Society, to welcome this fine volume celebrating the life and work of Hanna Segal under the able editorship of David Bell. The impressive and thoughtful group of contributors to this book, all distinguished psychoanalysts in their own right, each with his or her individual voice and emphasis, share in common their commitment to psychoanalytic thinking and their love and respect for Hanna Segal as psychoanalyst, colleague and friend. In the same spirit I warmly welcome the contributions to this most interesting work.

Irma Brenman Pick
President of the British Psycho-Analytical Society

Introductory Essay

Hanna Segal, the Work and the Person

The contributions collected in this volume form a tribute to Hanna Segal by some of those who have been profoundly influenced by her. It marks the first of two volumes, this first covering papers mainly on clinical and theoretical aspects of psychoanalysis, the second volume being mainly on applied work. This division is, though, rather artificial and confronted me with a problem. Hanna Segal, more than anyone else working within the Kleinian framework, has demonstrated the relevance of psychoanalytic ideas to human knowledge in general. Her papers on aesthetics, symbolism, and sociopolitical issues have made fundamental and original contributions which influence bodies of study far afield from psychoanalysis per se. Yet these contributions have not arisen from her 'setting about' applying psychoanalytic knowledge to other fields but have always been emergent from her immediate clinical and theoretical concerns. Her classic paper on aesthetics (Segal, 1952) can be read both as a clinical discussion of patients who have difficulties in their creative work and as a contribution to one of the central questions of aesthetics. Her study of Joseph Conrad (Segal, 1984) though on one level a psychoanalytic exegesis of his work, turns out to have immediate clinical psychoanalytic relevance as an examination of the roots of creativity in the depressive position and the relation of this to the mid-life crisis. Therefore, dividing the contributions to these volumes in this way should not be seen as reflecting a similar division in her work, which in fact shows a compelling unity. Langs quoted by Joseph in her introduction to *Dream, Phantasy and Art* (Segal, 1991), puts it pithily. Speaking of some of her papers he points out that they are not so much 'essays in applied psychoanalysis as an integral elaboration of her clinico-theoretical perspective'. So I hope this division can be seen as reflecting only the pragmatic needs of an editor.

Segal describes herself primarily as an artisan. By this she means that

1

the psychoanalytical problems that have arrested her attention have always arisen from the immediate exigencies of the practice of her 'craft'. Although many regard her as one of our leading theoreticians, she has always had some degree of suspicion of 'purely' theoretical problems. For her, a theory must show what it can do in the clinical situation and must address the primary material of the psychoanalyst's craft, the work with patients. This commitment to the clinical data is an important characteristic of Freud's. He did not allow theory to exist independently of his clinical observations and the latter were never sacrificed in the service of theoretical tidiness. Yet it is a paradox, though not a surprising one, that this attitude to theory is often just what underlies important theoretical developments and discoveries and this is certainly true of Segal. It links in my mind to her general attitude to intellectual endeavour; it must be something that emerges from the individual's interests and concerns. She has often pointed out that it is only by this route that original contributions are made in any field, coming about almost as a by-product of the compelling inner need to get to grips with a problem. Real originality emerges from that struggle, cannot be imposed upon it. The pursuit of originality as an aim in itself is bound to fail for this can only serve an illusory narcissistic ideal.

Psychoanalysis, perhaps more than any other discipline, is characterised by a dialectical unity between theory and practice. New observations compel the articulation of new techniques which in turn create the possibility of further new observations. This is clear in the history of the development of Freud's technique for example in the move from regarding the patient's feelings about the analyst as an unfortunate obstruction, to analysis of transference becoming a central focus of the work, which in turn yielded new phenomena of theoretical importance; or in Klein's discovery of the play technique opening the way to the observation of primitive mental states which necessitated new theories to house them. Segal's work exemplifies this tradition. Her work with psychotic patients and with artists blocked in their work led her to discoveries about the nature of symbolism and of the creative impulse, discoveries which in turn have opened the way to refinement of theory and technique. Segal, Herbert Rosenfeld, Wilfred Bion and Betty Joseph are the architects of that body of knowledge and research that forms the post-Kleinian development.

Biography

Hanna Segal (née Poznanska) was born in Lodz where her father had been sent on a political assignment for the nascent Polish Republic, but the family returned to Warsaw when she was three months old. Her father was a man of outstanding talents. His professional life spanned being a barrister, an editor of an international newspaper and the author of a classic work on French sculpture. He was also fluent in many languages. This combination of interests, both profound and broad, clearly had a deep effect on the direction of his daughter's interests. Her mother was an outstandingly beautiful woman but not at all vain. She had an enormous enthusiasm and zest for life. Although in Hanna's early childhood her mother led the life typical of a bourgeois lady, it was her resourcefulness and stamina that pulled the family through when they hit on very difficult times.

Hanna Segal's childhood was clouded by a deep trauma, the loss of her four-year-old sister Wanda, to whom she was deeply attached and who she remembers well, although she was only two and a half when she died. She did not go to school until 10 but once there enjoyed it tremendously. She flourished in the company of her schoolmates and so the move to Geneva, when she was twelve, was hard. However, she adored swimming in the lake and also learnt to row and ski. Swimming has remained a lifelong passion. She attended a very progressive international school which opened her mind to European culture but she remained attached to her roots and, when she was sixteen, her parents assented to her wish to return to Warsaw to complete her education.

Her deepest desire was to be a writer but she saw no point in dedicating herself to writing if she did not have faith in her capacity to produce great literature, so she resolved to study medicine. As she put it to me 'One of the things that attracted me to medicine was that I recognised that you could only produce something of lasting worth in literature if you had an extraordinary gift, whereas I realised that even with modest ability, without having to be first class, as a doctor you can do a reasonable amount of good just by doing your job'.[1]

She has always been, as she put it, 'an omnivorous reader'; the principal early intellectual influences were the 'continental' philosophers Voltaire, Rousseau, Montaigne, Schopenhauer and Nietzsche. It was, however, Pascal who particularly struck a chord with her and in adolescence she wrote an essay on one of his *Pensées*, 'Man is but a reed ... but he is a thinking reed'. Having recently reread her works I found myself returning again and again to this apparently simple aphorism as

3

it does capture an essential duality of life, that between internal and external. Man, like a reed, is blown by the winds of external circumstance but, unlike a reed, is never merely reactive to those circumstances in a passive way, he 'actively' apprehends them through the capacity for thought and, within limits, can act on those circumstances, changing them. A striking capacity to maintain a balanced perspective on this and the other great dualities that characterise life was to become one of the hallmarks of Segal's intellectual oeuvre.

By her late teens she had already read all of Freud that had been translated into Polish and also Laforgue and Pfister. The discovery of psychoanalysis at this time in her life was, as she put it, a 'a godsend'. It seemed to provide a basis for combining all her central preoccupations: her interest in the inner life as reflected in her love of literature, the wish to satisfy her social conscience and also, although she was perhaps not aware of it at the time, it gave expression to a highly developed scientific attitude to the world in general. However, when she asked Bychowski, the only psychoanalyst in Poland at the time, how to become a psychoanalyst he was entirely unhelpful, telling her she had to go to Vienna, which did not interest her in the slightest.

This period of her life was marked not only by her developing cultural interests but, seeing the extent of poverty and lack of political freedom, a more focused sociopolitical involvement. She joined the Polish Socialist Party. In the meantime the fascist President of Switzerland had expelled her father from Switzerland and both her parents, stateless and now moneyless, moved to Paris, where she joined them in 1939. Here she continued her medical studies and her political involvement, living in a flat which was a stop over for Spanish Republicans. Inevitably, the Spanish Civil war was the central preoccupation of all those whose sympathies were with the Left. In Paris she met the man she was to marry, Paul Segal, a mathematician who had a deep love of art and shared a lot of her cultural and sociopolitical interests.

In 1940, the beginning of the German occupation, the family had to take flight again and gained a passage to London on a Polish ship. In London Hanna re-established contact with some of her friends from Paris, one of whom was Kenneth Sinclair-Loutitt who whilst still a medical student had organised the ambulance service for the English contingent of the International Brigade. He introduced her to the circle of Left-wing intellectuals and writers of the 'Horizon' group, which included George Orwell, Stephen Spender and Cyril Connolly.

At first she was to continue her medical studies at the Royal Free Hospital, but the authorities insisted that she retake the exams she had already passed. However, some months later, Edinburgh University opened a faculty for Polish medical students which permitted her to continue her studies at the point where she had left off.

Edinburgh marked a watershed, for here she met Fairbairn to whom she has always felt indebted, both because he was her first real link to the psychoanalytic world and because of his neutrality. He told her how she could train and about the important debate going on in London. He gave her two books to read so that she might make up her own mind: Klein's 'The Psychoanalysis of Children' and Anna Freud's 'The Ego and the Mechanisms of Defence'. She read both and was immediately drawn to Klein. What struck her most was the vividness of the descriptions of the internal world of the child and Klein's capacity to capture the constant movement between internal and external. She was left in no doubt – she wanted to train as a psychoanalyst in London and be analysed by Melanie Klein and she set about this with determination.

For the time being however, she had to stay in Edinburgh to complete her medical education. Fairbairn introduced her to Dr David Matthews, a psychoanalyst who had been analyzed by Klein. He took her into analysis for the year until she moved to London. Her time with Matthews, though short, was very influential. She recalls that he walked with a noticeable limp and was quick to interpret her reluctance to notice it, or to explore its significance to her – the inevitable anxieties concerning the state of the primary object. In other words, he maintained an even respect for both internal and external reality.

The end of the next year brought her qualification in medicine, the end of her short time with Matthews and her move to London where she took a house job at Paddington Children's hospital. Following some insistence on her part she obtained a place in analysis with Klein but there was an immediate problem about the fee. The average fee was £1 per session, i.e. about £20 per month, exactly twice her monthly salary, but Klein suggested taking her on as a clinic patient. Whether she ever actually was a clinic patient is unclear as things were less formally organised then, but after 6 months she obtained a position at the newly established Polish Rehabilitation Centre where she got a proper salary and was then able to pay an ordinary fee. At that time mentally ill soldiers from the Polish army were admitted to Long Grove Hospital, one of the large mental hospitals outside London where conditions were generally appalling, especially for the Poles who spoke no English. Dr George Bram had been appointed to care for these patients and set his heart on getting as many as could out of hospital. He organised funds and appointed Hanna Segal as his second in command. Between them they established the rehabilitation centre which provided very good conditions and such treatment as they were able to organise. Here she learned a great deal about serious mental disorders, knowledge which influenced the direction of her psychoanalytic interests.

Segal's analysis with Klein was obviously the centre of her personal and intellectual development and she has commented elsewhere on her experience with Klein both as analyst and subsequently as supervisor and colleague (e.g. in the Klein centenary celebration at the Tavistock Clinic). The attributes that she particularly emphasised were Klein's professionalism, craftsmanship, psychoanalytic intuition and imagination, all firmly rooted within a strictly boundaried classical psychoanalytic setting. She was in analysis with Klein at the same time as Herbert Rosenfeld. It is worth remarking how Segal, Rosenfeld, and, much later, Wilfred Bion used their analysis with Klein to make scientific contributions which though obviously related are very distinct. This must be testament to Klein's capacity to allow her analysands to develop in their own ways.

The obituary to Klein, written jointly by Segal, Bion and Rosenfeld, emphasises Klein's commitment to truthfulness and quotes Samuel Johnson, 'Whether to see life as it is will offer us much consolation I know not; but the consolation which is gained from truth, if any there be, is solid and durable; that which may be derived from error must be, like its original, fallacious and fugitive'. Segal added that the search for truth is of course fundamental to all scientific endeavour but psychoanalysis is unique in that it is the capacity for truthfulness that is central to its therapeutic function.[2]

Early on in her analysis with Klein a particularly disturbing incident occurred, testament to the storm that was rocking the British Psycho-Analytical Society (of which she, of course, knew nothing). Her first admission interview was with Edward Glover, and things went reasonably well until he raised the issue of her needing to find a Training Analyst. When she said that there was no difficulty here as she already had a place with Klein, Glover got out of his seat saying there was nothing more to discuss and adding 'They train their own people'. In her next session she reported this adding angrily that there was something very mad going on. Klein must have been very shocked, but Segal remembers well Klein's capacity to protect her patient's analysis and how she avoided involving her in the political issues, something for which she was, eventually, very grateful. Klein explored her patient's view of what had happened, what it might mean, but also its significance for her in the ways it linked up with experiences from her own history.

6

Her supervisors during her psychoanalytic training were Joan Riviere and Paula Heimann, both of whom she respected greatly. She has always felt that Joan Riviere's stature has never been sufficiently recognised. Riviere, for Segal, was not only an outstanding clinician but an extraordinary intellectual with a broad and deep interest in literature and the arts . It was she who enlarged and deepened Hanna's knowledge of English literature and made her library available to her and Segal, for her part, introduced Riviere to Proust and Apollinaire.

She completed her psychoanalytic training in 1945 at the age of 27. The year 1946-7 was an extraordinary one as during it she married Paul, conceived her first child and presented her first paper 'A Psychoanalytic contribution to aesthetics' to the British Psycho-Analytical Society. She proceeded immediately to train as a child analyst being supervised by Paula Heimann, Esther Bick and Melanie Klein. In 1949 she read her membership paper 'Some aspects of the analysis of a schizophrenic'. She was appointed Training Analyst 5 years later. Ever since her qualification she has devoted her entire professional life to practising psychoanalysis, teaching and writing as well as holding numerous important positions within the British Psycho-Analytical Society including President, and on the international psychoanalytic scene, holding the position of Vice-President of the International Psychoanalytical Association on two occasions. In 1992, she was awarded the Sigourney award[3] for contributions to psychoanalysis.

Segal's Theoretical Contributions

In a work of this nature it is not possible to give a thorough appraisal of the substantial corpus of Segal's work both as an elucidator of Klein's ideas and as the author of those developments both in theory and technique that she has pioneered. Instead, I will focus on certain aspects which I think are central. It is also important to state here that Hanna Segal's contribution goes much further than her written work. Her contribution to scientific discussions, characterised by her ease in moving between the clinical and the theoretical, illustrating her position with apt clinical anecdotes and getting to the heart of the issue, have been very much part of the life blood of the British Psycho-Analytical Society.

In considering her theoretical contribution it is necessary to put it in historical context. The years between 1941 and 1945, during which Hanna Segal entered onto the scene, were those in which the British Psycho-Analytical Society was immersed in the political turmoil and debate known as the Controversial Discussions, which centred on Melanie Klein's discoveries (King and Steiner, 1991). It should be remembered that Freud had died only two years earlier and to some extent, opposing sides were preoccupied with the issue of what counted as a genuine development of his work and what represented a major deviation. This period not only generated a lot of heat but also shed considerable light as partisans of differing views were impelled to clarify their positions. This resulted in the presentation of papers that have remained seminal to the development of psychoanalysis in Britain. This was especially true of the paper by Susan Isaacs 'The nature and function of phantasy', (Isaacs, 1948). The issues raised in these discussions are not only of historical interest. They frequently resurface refracted through the lens of seemingly contemporary issues, for example in discussions of the therapeutic alliance, the 'real' relationship and the accessibility of deeply unconscious primitive phantasy. This is because the points of controversy go to the heart of our understanding of the psychoanalytic conception of the mind and the nature of the psychoanalytic task.

In 1946, the year after Segal's qualification, Klein published her groundbreaking paper 'Notes on schizoid mechanisms' (Klein, 1946) in which she described very primitive mental mechanisms that underlie serious psychopathological states. It was in this paper that she described clearly the splitting of the ego and the projection of parts of the self into objects, clarifying the anxieties and motives that underlie these processes. Her discoveries in this area provided the basis for her analysands Segal, Rosenfeld and subsequently Bion to carry this work forward through their treatment of psychotic patients. Rosenfeld, in 1947, described a borderline patient who developed a transference psychosis that he dealt with purely interpretatively and in the same year Segal presented her membership paper 'Some aspects of the analysis of a schizophrenic' which was the first report in the literature of a patient schizophrenic at the time of referral and treated without any fundamental alterations in classical psychoanalytic technique. In 1950 Bion presented his membership paper 'The imaginary twin' where he describes a psychotic aspect of the personality that 'goes back to the earliest relationship'.

One of the hallmarks of the Kleinian tradition is to be found in the relation between theory and practice. Theoretical formulations are always 'experience near' and some have seen this as a weakness of the theory, even a reification, believing it to make insufficient distinction between clinical descriptions of events, and models of mental function which are held to operate at a higher level of abstraction. For Klein and her followers this distinction does not hold and some would argue that it would not hold for much of Freud's theory either. This bridging between theory and clinical description was implicit from the start but was given its most elegant theoretical formulation in Susan Isaac's paper, referred to above.

Isaacs took the view, and this view has remained central to the present day, that the primary content of the unconscious is unconscious phantasy. Those processes we call mental mechanisms, such as projection, introjection, and identification are descriptions, so to speak, from the outside. From the inside, that is from the perspective of the subject, they are mentally represented by unconscious phantasy. Projection is associated with unconscious phantasies of the subject ejecting aspects of the self and object; introjection is associated with taking into the self aspects of the object which can then become identified with the self. These phantasies all ultimately depend upon the experience of bodily processes as the mind's perception of these bodily processes form the building blocks of all later psychological experience – as Freud (1923) put it 'the ego is first and foremost a bodily ego'. Wollheim (1969) has discussed the implications of this from a philosophical perspective. For him phantasies are the way that the mind represents to itself its own activities. These are not just representations, like a film going in parallel with the mental mechanisms, but it is a more unitary phenomenon, because the way the mind phantasises its own activities has crucial effects on the structure and functioning of the mind. For example the phantasy of projection, into objects of vital parts of the self, good or bad, often results in a feeling of emptiness. To some extent, this feeling arises from the mind's perception of its own state consequent on projection, it *really is* depleted.

My reason for focusing on this is not only that it is central to the Kleinian way of thinking about theory and clinical experience, but because I believe it is Hanna Segal who is its finest exponent. A striking characteristic of Segal's papers is her facility for using clinical examples that both vividly show the theory in action and pose problems which lead to further considerations of theory. This was used to great effect in her first book *Introduction to the Work of Melanie Klein* (1964), which has become a standard text. In this work she elucidates Klein's ideas demonstrating how they work in action, all the time bringing clinical examples of her own to illustrate theoretical points. Central to Segal's oeuvre is her study of the various manifestations of the depressive position, its link to symbolism and creativity and her development

9

of the understanding of the contents and functions of unconscious phantasy. As she put it to me 'My main interest is unconscious phantasy, the way it expresses itself, its relation to reality, internal and external, and its relation to perception'. Her extraordinary facility with dream material which occupies a central position in all her published papers bears testament to this.

'A psychoanalytic approach to aesthetics'

I would now like to use Segal's very first papers to illustrate some of these themes.

'A psychoanalytic approach to aesthetics' although not published until 1952 was in fact the first paper that Segal read to the British Psycho-Analytical Society in 1947, two years after she qualified. In this paper she brings together her psychoanalytic preoccupations with her involvement in art and literature. This paper was stimulated by her having in analysis psychotic patients and a number of artists who were blocked in their creative work. Both these groups of patients brought to the analysis fundamental problems with their capacity to use symbols freely. The blocked artists showed in the analysis a link between the paralysis in their work and their inability to mourn. This led Segal to explore the roots of creativity in the depressive position, and to develop a theory of aesthetics that, for the first time, provided a basis for understanding, from a psychological point of view, what it is about great art that makes it universal and enduring.

Freud's work in this area largely centred on two approaches: an exploration of the content of works of art in which he discovered universal themes, and an interest as to what infantile situations, from the artists own history, are reflected in the work. Such an approach could never answer the question as to how the artist achieves his effect upon his audience. An analysis based only on content would find similar themes in the great Greek tragedies and in evanescent pulp dramas and fails to distinguish between them. As Segal puts it, referring to earlier papers by Freud and others, 'They dealt with points of psychological interest but not with the central question of aesthetics, which is: What constitutes good art and in what essential respects is it different from other human works, from bad art in particular'.

Freud lacked adequate conceptual equipment for addressing this problem, though as is so often the case in Freud, this did not prevent him following his own intuition via a more literary, anecdotal route.

In 'On Transience' (Freud, 1916), written at the same time as he

10

wrote Mourning and Melancholia, he discusses a poet (who we now know to be Rilke) and a 'taciturn' friend who could not enjoy the beauty of their mountain walk because their awareness of its beauty was spoiled as it also brought awareness of the transience of life. This was not a problem for Freud. As he put it 'Transience value is scarcity value in time ... a flower that blossoms only for a single night does not seem to us on that account less lovely'. He agreed that awareness of all beauty must bring thoughts of death and the passing of all things but, as he pointed out, '... since the value of all this beauty and perfection is determined by its significance for our own emotional lives, it has no need to survive us and is therefore independent of absolute duration'. These considerations, however, had no effect on his friends which led him to the conclusion that a 'powerful emotional factor was at work' and he went on to describe this as 'a revolt in their minds against mourning'.

Segal puts the capacity to mourn, now enriched by Klein's elucidation of the inner struggle that forms the basis of the depressive position, both at the centre of the artist's work and of the audiences aesthetic response. Works of art derive their aesthetic depth from the artist's capacity to face the pain and guilt inherent in his perception of damage done to his good object and, through his creation of the work, to give substance to this struggle and to overcome it, the work itself being an act of reparation. We the audience are gripped by such works as we identify with the author's confrontation with the pain of his shattered internal world and obtain reassurance from his ability, through intense psychic work, to overcome it and depict it in his work of art.[4]

Segal draws on the French literature that had been so important to her in early adulthood – Proust, Flaubert and Zola. Proust made his observing of his need to write, and the functions it served for him, the basis of his work. He linked the creative work with the work of mourning describing a book as 'vast graveyard where on most of the tombstones one can read no more the faded names'. Segal describes how the artist, like the neurotic, suffers from all the pain and terror of a destroyed inner world but, unlike the neurotic, does not depend upon magical solutions. The artists has a highly developed awareness of the pain of his inner world but also the capacity to endure it and, through his equally highly developed reality sense,[5]gives form to his struggle, creating through it a real object which is always a communication to his fellow human beings.

Segal's patients could not bear the pain of these inner situations – like Freud's companions their minds revolted against mourning – and so were blocked not only in their artistic endeavours but also in other creative aspects of life, particularly in their sexuality. The incapacity to mourn appeared to arise from two principal sources: inability to bear the pain of guilt on the one hand, and, on the other intolerance of the separateness from the object that mourning inevitably brings, in other words for narcissistic reasons.

Segal reflects further both on the relation of form to content and on the nature of beauty, our love and terror of it. She points out that if beauty is the basis of one aspect of aesthetic experience then its contrary cannot be ugliness but only 'aesthetically indifferent'. Ugliness, being part of human experience often evokes aesthetic reactions that are in many ways similar to our response to beauty and Segal provides, through her model, a solution to this apparent paradox. Both beauty and ugliness together provide the aesthetic experience; in the great tragedies the ugliness is in the content whilst the beauty is in the form.

This paper has had a very wide influence far beyond the reaches of psychoanalysis but I will leave further discussion of it for the present.

'Some aspects of the analysis of a schizophrenic'

'Some aspects of the analysis of a schizophrenic' (Segal, 1950) was Segal's membership paper and was presented to the British Psycho-Analytical Society in 1949. I have already mentioned that this paper was a landmark in terms of treating such severe psychopatholgy and Segal contrasts her view with others particularly Federn and Fromm-Reichmann who had recommended major departures from ordinary technique in the treatment of these patients. These included the analyst attempting to nourish the positive transference, not interpreting the patients hostility and even going as far as to suggest that the analysis be interrupted if the transference becomes negative. In addition, this school held that defences and resistances should not be interpreted and that nothing should be brought into the patients consciousness that is unconscious 'as the ego of the psychotic is anyway submerged by it' (Federn, 1943). This position, I would suggest arose from two sources. Firstly, theoretically, it was assumed that the psychotic patient lacked the ego resources to manage any further anxiety and that understanding could not provide adequate containment. Secondly it is possible that this position reflects an unconscious capitulation to the extreme countertransference pressures which form an inevitable part of treating these patients.

Segal went into the analytic situation without these preconceptions – the ability of such patients to use psychoanalysis could only be worked

12

out in practice. 'My main aim was to retain the attitude of the analyst
... I tried to show him that I understood what he wanted from me, why
he wanted it so desperately ... I followed most interpretations (which
showed the patient that the analyst would not provide what he wished
for in action but through words) with an interpretation of what my
refusal had meant to him.' She pointed out that by not interpreting the
negative and destructive feelings and impulses the analyst would be in
fact reinforcing the profound splitting that lies at the root of the illness.
Also, the maintenance of an idealised and positive atmosphere was
likely to deflect the hostility elsewhere, with, from the patient's point
of view, the analyst's tacit support and most likely towards the members
of his own family, who would be ill equipped to deal with it. Her patient
tried desperately to recruit his analyst as an ally against his various
persecutors which included his doctors and various members of his
family. 'I thought it worthwhile in the analysis .. to attempt that which
Freud (1936) had shown to be the way of attacking the roots of a mental
illness, that is, not strengthening the defence mechanisms of the patient
but bringing them into the transference and analysing them'.

Edward, the patient, despite demanding all sorts of reassurances and
putting great pressure on his analyst to break boundaries, in the initial
stages, proved himself to be capable of using interpretations, to be
relieved by the understanding of his impulses and was not overwhelmed
by the bringing to consciousness of situations that were unconscious.
He depended very much on his analyst maintaining boundaries and
once when the analytic situation was fully established, revealed a dread
of his analyst giving into his pressure and thus confirming his omnipotence. He said one day, very anxious that she might overrun a session,
he having been late, 'You are my clock' (personal communication).

Although this is a very early paper, it does already demonstrate the
beginning of aspects of technique and clinical thinking that were to
become central to Segal's work. The patient, in the early stages, brought
a profusion of disjointed material but she was able to distil from this its
essence which consisted of two basic phenomena, which were connected (Bion, 1962a, was later to describe this as 'the selected fact').
These were the patient's preoccupation with a world that was destroyed
and his feeling of being changed. As Segal puts it 'he was afraid that the
world had been destroyed; he put a persecutory interpretation on what
had befallen him (he had not changed he had been changed); he seemed
unable to distinguish between himself and the world'.

Segal also raises in this paper an issue which has become a life long
preoccupation and which I will turn to shortly, namely the concrete

nature of the patient's experiences which she formulated as the patient's lack of capacity to distinguish between the symbol and the thing symbolised. He equated a 'stool' (as something to sit on) with stool (faeces) and 'stool' (the word).[6] She was to return to this fundamental issue. It is important to note that the patient was relieved by her pointing out to him that she understood that he did not feel able to make these distinctions so that feeling he was in prison and actually being imprisoned were the same thing. The implications of this are clear– for the patient to have understood this, there must have been an aspect of himself that was capable of making this distinction, otherwise the comment would have been meaningless to him.

When she describes the mechanism underlying hallucination she gives a striking example of the relation between theory and technique, showing how they are linked by the way she understands unconscious phantasy.

Edward suffered a major trauma: two male relatives died in quick succession. He remained superficially detached and described the second death as 'kind'. Segal points out that he was defending himself against the internalisation of terrifying persecuting dead and dying objects by saying in effect 'If I had such a (kind) death, I wouldn't be angry and come back and persecute people, and so I do not have to worry that he is angry and will persecute me'. Following a weekend he returned in a manic state, that, as the material revealed, involved triumphing over his dead objects which had then returned to persecute him. He described a buzz in his head, having to do eye exercises which were accompanied by counting and an echo which followed his counting. Segal clarified that the echo was mocking him and then elucidates the central mechanisms and unconscious phantasies. The counting was a typical obsessional mechanism, albeit experienced very concretely. It stood for his violent impulses against his objects (counting out a rival as in boxing) and, at the same time, served as a reassurance that good objects are still alive and intact as it also referred to counting the number of people in his family, counting the number of limbs.

The death of the two relatives had brought very primitive paranoid fears of the dead objects returning to persecute him internally, that he dealt with by disregarding them (counting them out). This was accompanied by feelings of triumph over them. Eye exercise were his way of using his eyes to invade and control objects that excluded him and which stimulated his curiosity (stirred up by the weekend separation), ultimately the primal couple. This invasion of the primal scene was felt also to annihilate the father as rival, thereby establishing unlimited

14

access to and control of his primary object.[7] However the objects that have been so attacked come to life internally and, filled with the patients own hating feeling, become the source of persecution and mockery (the echo).

In the next session he showed that things were getting a bit clearer as the buzz was now articulate and clearly said 'dreams dreams'. He subsequently described a dream which involved a fast game between people, a white man turning brown as he approached and he gave associations to films and photography. Segal saw this as confirming her interpretation. The filming and photographing represented his use of his eyes to invade the fast game (parental intercourse). She makes the point that the white man turning brown as he approached showed the phantasy contents of the mechanism of internalisation, i.e. as the man approaches, and is internalised for motives of control, he is turned to dangerous brown faeces which then become the source of persecution, controlling him (the patient) internally. The approaching man also stood for the patient's fear of an illness approaching. Segal took up this fear of a breakdown in the transference: the analyst, by showing the patient such a disturbing image of himself, that is making him aware of his illness, was experienced by the patient as the analyst concretely coming towards him and forcing illness, the hateful faeces, into him.[8]

> ... the dream gave us a link with the transference. As he tried to watch me in intercourse, while doing eye exercises, he swallowed me up in anger with his eyes and changed me into faeces. (He watches; they turn brown.) Then as the internal voice, I started persecuting him from the inside: "dreams, dreams". But reprojection occurs almost simultaneously. By looking, Edward also filled me with faeces; then, in retaliation, my looking both swallowed him up and changed him into faeces (by introjection) and filled him with faeces (by projection) so that, by looking at each other, we put excrements – illness and death – into each other.

Here Segal shows how mental mechanisms, as unconscious phantasies, alter both the nature of the objects and simultaneously of the ego. The man coming towards the patient and changing colour is viewed as the mind's representation of internalisation of an object carried out in anger.

The capacity to use material in this way, to relate it to primitive bodily phantasies that she both reconstructs in the transference and uses to lay out a corporealised mental geography, so well evidenced in this paper, became one of the hallmarks of all her later work.(Schafer's contribution in this volume discusses primitive bodily phantasies that underlie internalisation and 'blocked incorporation').

These reconstructions for Segal, are sometimes reconstructions of phantasies that do not bear a direct relation to actual events, whilst at other times they are re-enactments in the transference of real situations from the patients history. In a later paper (Segal, 1994) she describes a patient who had a repetitive dream of being persecuted by elongated animals with crocodile mouths, whilst he was tied to a chair. She noticed that he had a particular rigid posture and she was struck by the idea that he had been swaddled as a child and asked him if this was so. He confirmed this was indeed the case. He had been swaddled for four months and was told that he screamed in pain almost constantly. This, taken with the dream, gave the clue to a central characteristic of his personality – the constant feeling of being threatened.. His objects have, so to speak, had screamed into them his own perception of himself as a bound infant (the elongated bodies) with an enormous dangerous mouth. (The chapter by Brenman in this volume gives a very vivid example of this reliving in the transference of a similarly disturbing experience.)

Further Development of Segal's Work

Clearly, since these early papers, Segal's views have developed in a number of ways, but, as is often the case in the work of those who make such important contributions to knowledge, whether they be scientists or artists, early work prefigures the core of all later work. These two papers taken together bring the central concerns which were to dominate her contributions to both theory and technique in psychoanalysis, namely the nature of symbolic function, the elaboration and reconstruction of unconscious phantasy and the exploration of the roots of human creativity and destructiveness.

The paper on the treatment of a schizophrenic and various others that followed, demonstrated an expertise in treating psychotic patients, which in conjunction with the work of Bion, Rosenfeld and Henri Rey became central to this development of psychoanalysis. However, she has never liked to consider herself a specialist on psychosis, being rather wary of 'specialisms' of this sort, feeling they can lead to an overdramatisation, even romanticisation of the work. She said 'I only have one specialism and that is psychoanalysis'.

Segal has pointed out that although, theoretically, one might imagine that such patients are the most difficult to treat and the most demanding for the analyst, she has not found this always to be the case in practice. borderline patients often even more demanding. There are probably a variety of reasons for this. Segal has made the interesting suggestion that central to the difficulty in borderline cases is that there is always a catastrophe that is about to happen, and this hangs over the analysis as a constant threat. The patient may breakdown and it will be the analyst's fault and, as she has pointed out, this is in a certain sense true. With a schizophrenic patient, though confronted with difficulties of a different nature, the worst has already happened which to some extent allows the analyst more freedom to operate.

Segal discusses, also in this paper, another issue which formed the basis of further work, namely the problem of depressive anxiety in the psychotic situation. The patient felt that he was filled with insatiable greed and became preoccupied with the depletion of the world's food supply. She makes, here, an important phenomenological distinction: Although the phantasy is depressive in content (fears for the survival of his exhausted primary object), the feeling that accompanied it was persecutory.

'Depression in the schizophrenic'

She returns to the theme of depression in schizophrenia in her next published paper 'Depression in the schizophrenic' (Segal, 1956). Here she distinguishes different types of depressive state and, because the depressive situations were at first the object of violent projective procedures (as they could not be borne by the patient), she brings this together with a discussion of the countertransference.

Early in the analysis she was quite used to having to carry infantile feelings of rage and exclusion whilst her patient gave a dramatic evocation of herself involved in the primal scene. However, in a later session, although the patient skipped about gaily, as if scattering things, she felt a powerful feeling of sadness. Drawing on this atmosphere she was able to see that what the patient was scattering was her own depressive feeling, which included that consequent on awareness of her own illness. The patient, who was well read in literature, had previously, made numerous references to Shakespeare and it suddenly struck Segal that her patient skipping around gaily was just like Ophelia scattering her flowers. Her patient was scattering (projecting) her sad feelings into her analyst[9] who, like an audience watching Ophelia's mad behaviour in Shakespeare's play, had evoked in her these painful feelings. Using this intuition and the atmosphere of the session she was able to re-establish contact with her patient by putting her in touch with the sad feelings consequent on some progress in the previous days work.

This paper was read at the same congress as Bion read his 'Differentiation of the psychotic from the non-psychotic part of the personality' (1957) and Segal's patient, through her fragmenting and projective procedures, seemed to be using the same mechanisms that Bion described as underlying the formation of 'bizarre objects'.

At a point in the analysis where her patient felt more integrated she entwined threads of material in a way that was new. Previously she had broken such threads which seemed to represent her breaking of any trains of thought that might lead to awareness of depressive situations. The entwining of the threads gave form to a very poignant internal situation and she, the patient, said that there was something unbearable about it. Segal describes this as the patient having reclaimed both aspects of herself, her madness and her sanity (including her sane realisation of how ill she is). It was the holding both aspects of herself, keeping them in relation to each other which was so unbearable, as presumably was her awareness of her risk of confusing them. This again bears a striking similarity to Bion's description of the patient's fear that awareness of different parts of the self will not lead to integration but instead to the formation of a confusing unstructured conglomerate.

A preoccupation with the depressive position, a careful dissection of its vicissitudes, and an examination of the various manifestations of the anxieties and defences (particularly the manic ones) has remained at the core of Segal's work. She shows that the term 'depressive position' covers a wide variety of differing situations. Like Bion, she believes that clarifying these distinctions between different mental states (which though apparently subtle have profound implications) is in itself an important aspect of the therapeutic task. It is characteristic of her writing in general that she compares and contrasts situations that on the surface may appear similar but are, at a deeper level, in fact distinct. For example, she makes clear phenomenological distinctions between different types of persecutory situation. There is that arising from projection of vengeful parts of the self, characteristic of the paranoid-schizoid position, as opposed to the feelings of guilt which though characteristic of the depressive position, still have a persecutory quality. This would include stations where the object is recognised as damaged, responsibility is felt to lie with the self but the object is experienced as vengeful. There is also an acute form of mental pain sometimes present at the inception of the depressive position where the subject's awareness of his good object and the damage felt to have been done to it leads to guilt of a particularly omnipotent and persecuting kind.

These situations are quite distinct from the guilt and sadness, based on full awareness of separateness from the object, which release real reparative impulses.[10] In the former situations, where full separation from the object is not yet achieved, guilt can only be a source of persecution and tends to be dealt with either by denial or through masochistic sacrifice. The chapters by Anderson and Riesenberg Malcolm relate directly to this theme. Anderson describes a shift from a situation in which guilt is dealt with through further denial and destruction of the object that brings awareness of the depressive situation, to one where there is a capacity to bear real sadness. Riesenberg Malcolm describes a patient who felt so persecuted by his damaged objects that his only resort was to masochistic sacrifice or as she terms it, 'expiation'.

'Notes on symbol formation'

The next major development came with the publication of the paper 'Notes on symbol formation' (Segal, 1957). This paper elaborates further on a theme touched upon in her first paper and has become an enduring classic of psychoanalysis. In this paper she integrates a number of different lines of thought: the difference between symbolic and concrete thinking, the relation of symbolic function to the depressive position and the role of projective identification in symbol formation. She also brings to bear on the issue contemporaneous work on symbolism from other fields, namely that of the early semiotician Morris who pointed out that symbolic function involves a tripartite relationship the components of which are the thing symbolised, the thing functioning as the symbol, and the person to whom one represents the other. As Segal puts it 'In psychological terms, symbolism would be a relation between the ego, the object, and the symbol.' Her (now famous) patient said he did not want to play his violin because he didn't masturbate in public. Segal shows how calling this 'concrete thinking' doesn't really get us far as this might imply that the schizophrenic patient does not use symbols and this is obviously incorrect. He is clearly showing, at least from the observer's point of view, that the violin stands as a symbol for his penis. She compares the situation with a neurotic patient who dreamt that he and a girl were playing a violin duet and associations led to fiddling, masturbation etc. One might think that the crucial difference is that for the schizophrenic patient the symbol was conscious and for the neurotic patient it was unconscious but, as she points, out this does not suffice. When the neurotic patient becomes aware of the unconscious meaning of, for example, a paintbrush this doesn't usually have the effect of stopping him painting but, on the contrary may actually free him from a block. The crucial difference is not to be found in the psychic location of the symbol (i.e. conscious or unconscious) but in the way the symbol functions. In the patient who couldn't play his violin the symbol *is* formed but it is then equated with the thing symbolised so that he treats his violin, not as representing his penis, but concretely as his penis, a situation which Segal describes as forming a 'symbolic equation'.

This has important implications for technique in that patients who function in this way also treat words as being the things they represent (as with Edward, the patient referred to above who equated the word 'stool' with actual faeces) and so may react to the analyst's words as if they were acts. Segal goes on to show that the transition to 'symbolism proper' is an important outcome of the move towards the depressive position. Sohn's Chapter in this volume discusses a particularly disturbing outcome of the failure to symbolise where acts of violence are in themselves symbolic equations.

The difficulty of the patient who forms these 'symbolic equations' arises from his use of projective identification.[11] When parts of the ego and its objects are projected into an object which ordinarily would stand as a symbol, the resulting confusion between ego and object results in the symbol becoming 'the thing itself'. When this confusion is overcome, so that ego and object are differentiated, the symbol can stand for the thing symbolised but also retain qualities of its own and is thus distinct from the original object. Caper's Chapter elaborates further Segal's contribution in this area as well as its relation to her work on creativity.

Other Aspects of Hanna Segal's Work

I would like now to turn to some other aspects of Segal's work which have been influential. I am referring to her conceptualisation of the nature of the psychoanalytic task, her focus on the capacity for realistic perception of the internal and external world, and her clinical elaboration of Freud's and Klein's formulation of the death instinct.

To turn firstly to the nature of the analytic task and its therapeutic value. On this Segal is clear, her viewpoint is very classical. Conflict is at the centre of the psychoanalytic conception of mind and the improved mental health to be gained from psychoanalysis is based on the acquisition of insight into these conflicts. All of psychoanalytic technique subserves this basic aim. She discussed this at some length in a paper given to a symposium and subsequently published (Segal, 1962). Her view is clearly linked to what she had said in the obituary of Klein, mentioned above, where she focused on the mind's capacity for truthfulness as central to psychic health.

So why is insight therapeutic? She offers the following considerations. First insight is therapeutic because it leads to the regaining and integration of lost aspects of the personality, allowing, therefore, a normal growth of the personality. This reintegration of the ego allows the object to have its own characteristics, as distinct from those which have been projected into it, and so is inevitably accompanied by a more accurate perception of reality, external and internal. Second insight is therapeutic because knowledge replaces omnipotence and therefore enables a person to deal with his own feelings and the external world in more realistic terms.

Other contributors at the symposium discussed the issue of analysis as a 'corrective experience', a conception that carries with it the implication that the analyst makes up for deprivations in the patient's past through the use of special techniques that go beyond that provided by the classical psycho-analytic setting. For Segal psychoanalysis *is* a corrective experiences *as classically practised*. To paraphrase her, projecting aspects of oneself or one's internal objects into an analyst who doesn't identify with them nor react to them, but who can really think about them, is a corrective experience. It helps the patient become aware of himself and distinguish phantasy from reality. Special techniques which involve the analyst in becoming a 'good' object for the patient cannot be therapeutic as they will collude with splitting processes which alienate the patient from himself. In addition, such techniques may make the patient feel that the analyst cannot tolerate being a 'bad' object and this is an important consideration. Psychoanalysts choose their profession at least partly out of wishes to repair damaged internal objects (which has to be distinguished from the determination to control them). It is important however that the analyst can tolerate the presence of an object that cannot be repaired, allow himself to be perceived as bad without either sinking into despair or retaliating whether with hostility or excessive therapeutic zeal. Manoeuvres to secure a positive transference clearly evade this struggle.

Similar considerations apply to the question of the 'therapeutic alliance' and the 'real relationship'. Segal prefers the more ordinary word 'co-operation' as the term 'therapeutic alliance' again brings with it associations with particular techniques aimed at securing such an alliance, not through understanding, but through more manipulative means. For Segal, the reality of the analyst is of great importance. It is vital that the patient feels that his analyst can tolerate the patient's perception of him, particularly when these are realistic, but this has to be combined with the analyst's capacity to explore the significance of these perceptions for the patient (as for example in Matthew's exploring with Segal the meaning to her of his limp, or Klein's way of handling Segal's first brush with the furore of the Controversial Discussions).

Discussion of the 'real relationship' often gets polarised between those who seem to imply that it is not what the analyst *says* but who he *is* that counts, and those who can appear to imply that it is only the interpretations that matter. In characteristic style Segal goes right through the centre of the horns of this false dilemma. Of course who the analyst is, his character and his strengths and weaknesses, is important, but it is through his capacity to say what he says and in his way of saying it that the analyst *shows* the patient who he is.

Some writers use Bion's theory of 'container-contained' to underwrite a conception of the analyst's task that can at times appear over concrete. The analytic work becomes 'containing' the patients projections and metabolising them as if replacing and making up for the mothers failures in infancy. Segal is very wary of this on a number of points. Firstly it does not adequately distinguish between psychoanalysis and mothering, secondly, it makes it appear that the curative factors are coming only from the analyst rather than from the patient, and both of these combined easily lead to an unfortunate analytic grandiosity.

For Segal, the principal factors that lead to change are to be found in the patient himself. The analyst supports the patient in rediscovering his own developmental possibilities which have become arrested. Her view is very close to that put forward by Strachey in his seminal paper (1934). He showed that whenever the analyst makes a full interpretation in the transference he is at one and the same time acknowledging his status as an archaic object in the patient's world and differentiating himself from such objects. There is always a pressure to become the 'real' object for the patient but he points out that this is more complex than might at first appear to be the case.

> The analytic situation is all the time threatening to degenerate into a 'real' situation. But this actually means the opposite of what it appears to. It means that the patient is all the time on the brink of turning the real external object (the analyst) into the archaic one; … In so far as the patient actually does this, the analyst becomes like anyone else the patient meets in real life– a phantasy object.

Segal also places emphasis on reconstruction in two senses. Firstly, the reconstruction of unconscious, and ultimately bodily, phantasies and secondly, of the importance of the understanding of the reliving in the transference/countertransference situation of real events of the patient's infantile past such as parental illness, traumatic separations, births of siblings (she has always held the view the birth of a sibling before there is the mental capacity to deal with it, has profound effects on the developing personality, sometimes of a psychotic kind.) Sandler and Sandler discuss further the question of reconstruction in their chapter.

The stress within the Kleinian tradition of the importance of a clear understanding of the transference is often misunderstood and turned into a sort of empty technical procedure. This degrading of a good idea into mechanical procedures is a common process. Tom Main (1968) called it the move from possessing an idea (an ego function) to becoming possessed by it (a superego function). In the latter case transference interpretations become a sort of fetish object. Making interpretations that contain reference to the analyst's person are used as if having some magical significance. Segal often refers to this as the 'also ran' interpretation. She likens the analyst's applying, mindlessly, to himself anything that the patient attributes to various people or situations in his life, to a racing commentary which always lists those that 'also ran'. The issue for Segal is not transference interpretations *per se* but a clear understanding of the patient, and his difficulties. She holds with Freud and Klein that the patient's difficulties cannot be dealt with '*in absentia*' so that a deep understanding of the transference situation (or as Betty Joseph puts it 'the total situation') is central but this has to be distinguished from interpretations themselves being applied as an empty technique.

This deeper understanding of the transference is reflected in O'Shaugnessy's contribution to this volume where she shows how patient and analyst may use a misunderstanding of the transference to turn the analysis into an enclave where the patient feels protected from all the problems of living.

Segal, like Klein, has taken very seriously Freud's theory of the death instinct though she has always preferred, the French term 'pulsion' which gives it a more psychological quality. She has made it a clinically relevant concept. For, her the death instinct 'only has meaning in its perpetual conflict with the life instinct' (Steiner, 1997). Segal has shown two principal ways in which the death instinct shows itself. In one situation, easier to see as it is so overt, it manifests itself as a hatred of life and living, this being linked to Freud's (1915) model of the ego's 'primordial repudiation of the external world'. She illustrates this with Jack London's story 'Martin Eden'. Martin who is drowning finds himself automatically attempting to swim, and he shows his own hatred of his instinct for survival 'This is the will to live he thought, and the thought was accompanied by a sneer'.[12] The second situation is more pervasive and less easily defined, its expression mirroring its content as a silent lure towards a deadly passivity which is idealised. Segal has also pointed out that awareness of such terrible destructiveness often re-leases powerful reparative forces and that such awareness, therefore, has an important relation to creativity in general. As she puts it in her 1947 paper discussing the question of aesthetics:

> ... ugliness-destruction-is the expression of the death instinct; beauty-the desire to unite into rhythms and wholes– is that of the life instinct. The achievement of the artist is in giving the fullest expression to the conflict and the union between the two.

Another aspect of Segal's approach, which has acquired increasing importance to her is her focus on perception. It relates directly to her conception of the analytic task as helping the patient to see things clearly and differentiate himself from his objects. Clear vision of the internal and external situations is one of the aims of the whole psycho-analytic endeavour. Segal holds with the view that we have an inbuilt 'grammar of object relations' whose expression is infinite (she models this on Chomsky's theory of a universal syntactic structures) and which we use to explore the real world and discover it.

In closing this section it might be helpful to touch on the ways that Hanna Segal sees her work as having developed. Bion has been the major influence. This is clear from the first volume of her previously published papers where she adds postscripts to indicate the directions her thinking has taken and, in almost every case, she makes mention of Bion's work. She makes particular use of Bion's model of the 'container-contained' and on his distinction between normal and pathological forms of projective identification. She draws on both these ideas to enrich her theoretical perspective,[13] and in terms of their implications for analytic technique. Here I am particularly referring to the shift in emphasis towards examining the way the patient and analyst enact aspects of the patients internal situation so that phantasy of projective identification is 'actualised' (Sandler, 1976).

In the postscript written to her 1954 paper 'Notes on schizoid mechanism underlying phobia formation' she looks back at the clinical material with the advantage of 25 years further experience: 'I think I completely failed to analyse the transference properly. Her projective identification was not just a phantasy; I seem to have been quite unaware of the way in which it was happening in these sessions ...Today I would been more concerned with showing her what she was actually doing in the session in the moment to moment interaction between us. I would concentrate less on the detailed content of her phantasies and dreams.'

Although she puts stress, therefore, on the way the analyst can be 'stage managed' by the patient into playing a particular part she has always remained cautious as there is an easy slippage into making a virtue of necessity and idealising enactments. From Segal's point of view these enactments are inevitable in the practice of psychoanalysis and much is learnt from them but she maintains a more classical perspective. The capacity of the analyst to be the recipient of intense and disturbing states of mind, to really experience the experiences and to think about them without enactment remains that which we aim, however imperfectly, to achieve.

I am reminded here of a famous comment of Klein's at a scientific meeting of the British Psycho-Analytical Society. An analyst had presented material in which he had made a serious mistake from which he and the patient had learnt a great deal and then went on rather to recommend the making of mistakes, making a virtue of necessity. Klein said, ironically, that she admired this analyst whose work was of such a high order that he worried about not making mistakes. She found that she made quite enough mistakes in every analytic hour without having to bother about facilitating it. Or as Segal has put it 'We learn a lot from mistakes but the less there are the better the work'.

In the postscript to the symbolism paper, written in 1979, she links her theory of symbolic function directly with Bion's model of 'the container-contained'. For some patients the difficulty in symbolisation, resulting in a drive towards enactment and concrete gratification, arises from an infantile traumatic situation where the mother, for reasons of her own, was not able to contain adequately and manage the infants projections. In other patients this appears not to have been the case. She describes two patients one of whom was compromised by his experience of an object which was never felt to manage his projections and instead forcibly reprojected frightening contents into him. The other patient appeared to have a profound envy of the capacity of her object to manage and sought to strip it of this quality. Of course, one can never really know in any absolute sense exactly what happened in childhood (powerful envious impulses sometimes arise from deprivation and at other times seem to be the cause of it) but, for Segal it is important to be able to think about these distinctions and clarify them as far as one can.

The relationship between the container and the contained is in health one that is mutually satisfying and growth promoting . Segal in a later paper on symbolism (Segal, 1978) describes a situation where this relation is one of mutual emptying and stripping of all meaning. In this situation the patients use of words as symbols was profoundly disturbed. (Brenman's chapter describes a less disturbed patient in whom however this pathological relation between container and contained was at times a central feature of his psychopathology.)

Segal's stress on the tripartite nature of symbolism has brought important links with the oedipal situation, which Bion and others have subsequently developed. Segal has described how in the analytic situation there is an inherent triangularity – the analyst, the patient and the words. Some patients who feel the need only for action regard the demand for words as an intrusion into a phantasied relationship with the primary object who is felt (through projection) to know them without having to be told in words. In her introduction to *The Oedipus Complex Today* (1989) she comments on Britton's (1989) chapter which describes a triangulated mental space made up of the patient, his relationship to individual parental figures, and the relationship between the parental figures which excludes him but which he observes. Segal, again emphasising the bodily unconscious phantasies, points out that the triangle whose sides are made up of these different relationships does not enclose an empty space but implicitly creates a space in which a new baby might find its place.

In fact Segal had already linked the primitive oedipal situation to the capacity for symbolism in her early work. One of the patients described in the aesthetics paper was blocked in her ability to write and discovered that she hated words. She said that using words made her break 'an endless unity into bits'. This endless unity referred to the phantasy of total possession of the primary object. As words were felt to disrupt this phantasised unity, they were felt, concretely, as violent intruders forcing upon her mind awareness of separateness from her objects, and this underlay her being blocked in her ability to write.

This preoccupation with projective identification and enactment is also the basis of Segal's important work on the function of dreams (Segal, 1980). Here she distinguishes those dreams which serve to communicate something to the dreamer and through him to the analyst, from those dreams that primarily serve the function of evacuation of unwanted psychic contents. Segal lays particular stress on the way dreams demonstrate unconscious insight . I will quote in full a particularly interesting example of Segal's work with dreams which unites a number of the themes I have touched on– the dream as communication of unconscious insight, the confusion of phantasy and reality, and the relation of the omnipotent destruction of the capacity to think to the oedipal situation.

The patient though not psychotic suffered from hallucinations. In one session he commented that 'there was no guard at the door' and there followed excited sexual material accompanied by the thought 'I can do what I want'. He went on to tell the following dream.

> I was explaining to M (his girlfriend) about my hallucinations. I was telling her 'Look, I dream up a car and there it is' And the car appeared. He got into the front seat. But there was no partition between front and back – no pole to lean against. He started falling backwards, feeling an utmost panic. And he awoke with severe anxiety.

Segal points out that 'pole' is a condensation of a phallic symbol, his Polish analyst and her husband's name (known to the patient) Paul. In the absence of the father/penis/ analytic function there is nothing to stop him from having intercourse completely unrestrained with the analyst/mother. But it also means access to unrestrained projective identification with loss of all boundaries confusion and panic.

What he seems to explain in the dream is that his 'ability' to make his thoughts realities and so control the world, is in unconscious phantasy, the projection of himself into his primary object (the world for the infant) destroying all boundaries. The important development is that the whole process, instead of giving rise to hallucination, on this occasion achieved representation in a dream. Subsequent to the work on this dream the patient's hallucinations disappeared.

The development of Segal's work on enactment has been has been also very influenced by Betty Joseph who has made the detailed study of subtle shifts between communication and acting the centre of her work. She demonstrates this very vividly in her paper in this volume where she links enactment to Segal's interest in the function of perception.

Hanna Segal: The Person

I would like to end this introductory essay by making a few comments about Hanna Segal on a more personal level. Her enthusiasm and zest for life are testament to the fact that awareness of the depths of human destructiveness does not impart a pessimistic outlook. For her there is no division between psychoanalysis and life and she would agree with those philosophers who see psychoanalysis not as a special theory derived from and relating to particular practises that take place within the peculiar circumstances of a psychoanalytic session, but as an extension, though a very profound one, of the understanding human beings have of each other, a way of explaining what that understanding is and how it comes to be.

I first met Hanna Segal as supervisor of my first training case. At that time I was rather overanxious to be psychoanalytically 'proper', to maintain neutrality which meant as I saw it being rather adept at side-stepping the numerous invitations my patient made for me to 'act in' with her. Segal clearly thought I was being overfussy and said to me 'You cant do this work, you know, without getting your boots dirty. If you do, you can always clean them off afterwards'. This made an abiding impression on me. I said above that Segal is cautious lest understanding the inevitability of enactment leads to a casualness in technique. Here however she also showed me the dangers of a refusal to be involved.

During my many years of supervision and subsequent participation in her clinical seminar I have been struck again and again by her capacity to maintain balance between internal and external situations, between good and bad, theory and practice, reality and phantasy. She also has an extraordinary capacity to hear extremely disturbing and perverse material without becoming judgmental, managing to maintain a keen interest. What can this mean? What are the unconscious and infantile phantasies that are being brought? What comes over more than anything is her deep conviction about the value of psychoanalysis and the importance of truthfulness.

Of course, very evident is her ability to see and reconstruct bodily phantasies from the material. She is as she put it 'a very bodily sort of person' and she always tries to have in her mind a kind of bodily map of the patients mental functioning, though not necessarily choosing to interpret to the patient in those terms. In one seminar we were discussing another analyst's patient, who was very ill. He was the oldest of a large Irish family and before he was a year old his first sibling arrived, to be followed by 6 others in quick succession. The analyst had shown how whenever he made contact with the patient the patient immediately transformed this into an experience of violent intrusion. He brought a dream about being given white medicine which was wonderful but then became disgusting. Associations led to phantasies of buggery.

Segal brought this together. Every time the patient felt understood he experienced it as contact with a good maternal breast which immediately became contaminated with father's semen turning feeding into a poisonous assault. She linked this to the fact that when he was less than three months old his mothers mind was so to speak, already contaminated with the new baby, fathers semen, which was felt to have intruded in a hateful way. This of course was further compounded by the arrival of four more siblings at short intervals.

Segal brings to bear her very wide reading and can often find a fitting story or anecdote to capture the essence of a situation. One of my patients a very disturbed middle-aged woman, made unceasing demands on me to extend sessions, to have sessions over weekends etc. Having projected important aspects of her own ego functions into me, she found breaks intolerable (she regarded weekend breaks as being guillotined) and the danger was very real. This process resulted, eventually, in her having to be admitted to hospital where I continued her analysis. Inevitably there were many people involved in her treatment and she always seemed to be recruiting others who often telephoned me. There were psychiatrists, nurses, social worker, GP and an occupational therapist.

I learnt that all of the people involved in her care were having a meeting but they accepted that I wouldn't be attending. This made the patient very upset and her demands escalated. I had understood her demand for me to attend the meeting as yet another attempt to involve me in hours outside her sessions but found I was reaching an impasse. Segal though sympathetic to my dilemma and the approach I was taking, picked up something more desperate in the atmosphere. She recalled a poem by Appolinaire who imagined all the people he had known coming together and building a pyramid that made him whole. This led us to see that the patients dilemma was that she projected so massively into her various carers that she felt the only way she could become integrated was, concretely, through the meeting of those in whom these aspects of herself were lodged. My not attending the meeting, therefore, made her feel that an essential element, those aspects of her which she felt were located in me, would be absent from the meeting and this made her feel increasingly desperate. This understanding freed up the situation considerably.

On another occasion I discussed a patient who brought material about attending his parents wedding anniversary celebration. Various relatives asked him how he was and he said he was 'OK' which he knew was what his parents wanted him to say (so he protected his parents' celebration). He claimed, however, that this was pure hypocrisy on his part as he didn't really care about the party, was only pretending to be concerned to protect it etc.. It reminded Segal of one of Montaigne's aphorisms 'Hypocrisy is the homage vice pays to virtue'. In other words the hypocrite who only gives an affectation of virtue is still showing through his act that he does know what virtue is.

Segal is a compulsive reader and at one time she had a great interest in science fiction. She particularly liked those writers who could create imaginary worlds and then work out what would happen in such a world. This interest links with the way she has described the use of phantasy and imagination which can be like 'hypotheses' about the world. 'What would happen if such and such was the case'.[14] I once asked her if she found her broad literary knowledge helpful in her analytic work. She replied that all ones life experiences influence ones work – ones experience of relationships, having children and so, of course her, literary interests, like all her other experiences, had their influence. She would be extremely wary of using literary allusions in her clinical work unless there were very good grounds for doing so, such as their being already clearly present in the patients material. In the example of the schizophrenic who was scattering aspects of herself like Ophelia scattering flowers, she would not have directly referred to Ophelia if she had not known that the patient was so involved in her mind with Shakespeare's plays.

Although keenly interested in the countertransference it would be unusual for her to ask an analyst what he felt during the session, though she is always attentive to the atmosphere and equates the openness of the analyst to be affected and involved emotionally with his patient to Freud's free floating attention – i.e. it is not just an openness to thoughts but also to feelings. Segal has remained somewhat cautious of the use of countertransference as it can so easily become a misuse. As she has often put it 'Countertransference can be the best of servants, but is the most awful of masters'. I don't think she would hold with interpreting the countertransference to the patient unless it is already clearly indicated in the patients material.

She has a peculiar knack of getting to the heart of things and has a deep aversion to 'padding,' something that is clearly demonstrated in her written work. Her lively sense of humour is also an essential part of her character, which she can also use to good effect.

In the same way that she brings her own life experiences to the psychoanalysis she brings her analytic sense to many other situations. Some time ago there was an important political meeting of the British Psycho-Analytical Society. The question at issue was whether or not to pursue our participation in the conferences of the UKCP (a broad umbrella organisation set up to form a register of the various psychotherapies including a plethora of widely differing theories and techniques). At a previous meeting it had been agreed that the Society would agree to continue to participate provided that a number of specific proposals that we put forward were accepted. A speaker pointed out that ninety-five per cent of the Society's proposal had been agreed and this was a great success. We should not be bloody minded about what had not been accepted as it amounted to only five per cent.

Hanna Segal took the podium and said that it all depended which five per cent it was. In this case it referred to training requirements for psychoanalytic psychotherapists. She said she was reminded of a patient in analysis with her who had great difficulties in her relationships with men. She recently met a man and extolled all his virtues and was planning to marry him. She pointed out that he was kind, intelligent, shared her cultural interests, was fun to be with etc. She went on to say that there was only one small problem which she didn't think mattered. She, so to speak, was not going to make this a sticking point – he was impotent. Segal went on to say that it may be 'just five per cent' but that five per cent happens to be the balls of the matter and agreement to leaving it out would amount to an act of self-castration.

Her interest in politics has remained abiding, her sympathies remain with the Left although she has not engaged in overt political activity for most of her professional career. However, she became so convinced of the real danger of the widespread denial of nuclear threat in 1980's that she felt that saying nothing about it amounted to a collusion. She co-founded, with Moses Laufer, the organisation of Psychoanalysts for the Prevention of Nuclear War (PPNW) in 1983. Apart from its organisational and political work, linking up with other anti-nuclear organisations the PPNW was responsible for an important body of work examining from a psycho-analytic perspective the nuclear threat, the role of secrecy, and the various psychic defences that function to evade the reality of the nuclear threat. Her paper 'Silence is the real crime' takes its title from a passage in the book 'Hope against Hope' by Nadezhda Mandelstam. Her husband, the poet, Osip Mandelstam was hounded by the Stalinists and sent to the gulag. Nadezhda Mandelstam wonders as to what our reaction should be to such horrors. She does not side with those who think we should be noble about it, facing our death with quiet dignity. She call upon us to side with the cow which, on its way to slaughter, screeches, bellows and kicks. This, for Mandelstam, is the more human response. We should scream and hope that maybe somewhere, someone may hear for as she puts it 'Silence is the real crime'.

Segal's paper is also making the point that one aspect of mental health is our ability to really engage with the world about us and, as individuals, be able to resist collusion with the various myths that society and its rulers create for our comfort.

Following the end of the cold war Segal (1995) drew attention to the danger of the 'manic triumphalism' of the Western ideologues who now felt they could rule the world with no obstacles in their way. She anticipated the need to find a new enemy both to justify the continuation of the arms industry (the external factor) and (the internal factor) out of a need to find an external object to be hated, so deflecting attention from any awareness of responsibility for the misery, unemployment and poverty 'at home'. Such an enemy was soon found in Saddam Hussein.

As a final anecdote which illustrates her capacity to maintain common sense, a perhaps underrated quality in the practice of psychoanalysis, I want to relate an event that took place in a clinical seminar some years ago. The patient being discussed was a single mother whose daughter, a child of 7, was in analysis. She had a steady relationship with a man but had decided not to live with him. She had however conceived a child who had just been born. She felt she would have to stop the other child's analysis and gave a number of important reasons as to why it wasn't practicable to take the child to her sessions.

The seminar divided into two. One group, identified with the child in analysis, pointed out that the arrival of the new sibling, a considerable trauma for her, meant that it was now even more important than ever that she continue her analysis. The other group, identified with the mother, pointed out how impossible it was for her to get her daughter to analysis having now a small baby to take care of. Segal, after listening to this debate which was getting more and more animated, if not rather self-righteous said: 'Well, it is true that the child now needs her analysis more than ever, but maybe its a sad fact that it may not be possible for her to have it.'

I bring this anecdote as it shows what I think is central to Hanna Segal both in her work and as a person and that is her ability to maintain a balanced perspective. Richard Wollheim, at the launch of her last book, chose this capacity for balance as his main theme. He had in mind her consideration of the life promoting and destructive forces in the human mind. In this introductory essay I have had cause to mention various other polarities which she has approached with the same balanced outlook – such as that between theory and technique, internal and external, phantasy and reality, environment and constitution. Her heritage provided her with a deep love of all things human but most especially those two great pillars of human achievement which I believe she so well embodies, and which gave me the title for this book: *Reason and Passion*.

Notes

1. This and similar quotations are from interviews conducted with Hanna Segal in November 1995.

2. She has on various occasions carefully drawn the distinction between 'truth' with a small 't', more a function of truthfulness, from 'Truth' with a capital 'T', absolute truths, which bear all the hallmarks of omniscience and arrogance.

3. The Mary S. Sigourney Trust set up the Sigourney Award for outstanding contributions to psychoanalysis. The award rotates between the continents and Segal was among the first Europeans to receive it.

4. Freud in 'On Narcissism' (1915) touches on the need to create something in order not to fall ill. He wonders why man ever leaves the satisfactions of his narcissistic state to face all the pain of the struggle with the real world. His theory could not provide an answer but he found one in the work of the poet Heine's 'picture of the psychogenesis of creation': God is imagined as saying 'Illness was no doubt the final cause of the whole urge to create. By creating I could recover, by creating I became healthy'.

5. The reality sense is particularly clearly seen in the artist's respect for his materials and the technical aspects of his work, his knowledge of their powers and their limitations and also of course the artist's full appreciation of internal reality.

6. She also makes the interesting point that he at other times showed a difficulty which was the converse. Instead of being overwhelmed by the symbolic meanings of objects he experienced the objects as devoid of any meaning at all. As she puts it 'the unconscious equation remained unchanged but consciously the symbolism had to be completely denied. A cigarette was just a cigarette …'

7. Segal has described similar mechanisms as central to mania, i.e. the feeling of invasion and possession of the primary object, all obstacles, standing psychically for the father, being destroyed – which of course shows the link between mania and paranoia.

8. This description in effect anticipates Bion's model of the outcome when projective identification is not contained by the object (mother/analyst) but instead violently reprojected into the baby/patient.

9. Discussion of countertransference and its relation to projective identification, now very much part of the contemporary psychoanalytic scene was very novel at this time. It was only a few years before this paper was originally presented that Heimann's paper 'On countertransference' (1950) first gave full articulation to the idea of countertransference not just being a problem of the analyst but also being a communication from the patient. Segal has remained cautious in her application of this to the clinical situation and I will discuss this below.

10. Klein's supervisees (in a radio programme some years ago) stressed the emphasis she put on locating and distinguishing the real depressive situation in the material. She would point out that in some patients even a fleeting reference awareness of the goodness of his object should not be missed. Describing the patient's feelings of persecution and hostility was all very well but missing a patient's reference to his good feelings for his object was regarded as a costly oversight as it is here that the analyst can find his real ally.

11. Although Segal is using the same term as Klein it clearly has different referents and she was later to agree with Bion in distinguishing normal from pathological types of projective identification.

12. This has obvious links with Rosenfeld's work (1971) where he describes the patient being drawn into a destructive world where the 'libidinal' and needy parts of the self that are struggling towards a good object, are cruelly mocked.

13. Segal has remarked 'It is an obvious truism that the environment is of fundamental importance but until Bion's work we had no adequate model of how the environment exerts its importance'.

14. She has elsewhere drawn the distinction between imagination used for 'What if?' as opposed to a different situation where this vital function degenerates, becoming a world of 'As if'.

References

Bion, W.R. (1950) 'The Imaginary Twin' in Bion, W.R. (1967), *Second Thoughts*. London: Heinemann.

—— (1957)'Differentiation of the psychotic from the non-psychotic personalities', *International Journal of Psycho-Analysis*, 38; 266-75. Repr. in Bion, W.R. (1967), *Second Thoughts*. London: Heinemann.

—— (1962a) *Learning from Experience*. London: Heinemann.

—— (1962b) 'A theory of thinking', *International Journal of Psycho-Analysis*, 43: 306-10. Repr. in Bion, W. R. (1967), *Second Thoughts*. London: Heinemann.

Federn, P. (1943) 'Psychoanalysis of psychosis', *Psychiatric Quarterly*, 17: 3-19.

Freud, S. (1914) 'On Narcissism: an Introduction' *S.E.* 14

—— (1915) 'Instincts and their Vicissitudes' *S.E.* 14

—— (1916) 'On Transcience', *S.E.* 14.

Heimann, P (1950) 'On counter-transference', *International Journal of Psycho-Analysis*, 31:81-4.

Isaacs, S. (1948) 'The nature and the function of phantasy', *International Journal of Psycho-Analysis* 29: 73-97.

King, P. and Steiner, R. eds, (1991) *The Freud-Klein Controversies*. London: Routledge.

Klein M. (1946) 'Notes on some schizoid mechanisms', *International Journal of Psycho-Analysis*, 27: 99-110.

Rosenfeld, H.A. (1947) 'Analysis of a schizophrenic state with depersonalisation', *International Journal of Psycho-Analysis*, 28: 130-9.

—— (1971) 'A clinical approach to the psychoanalytic theory of the life and death instincts: an investigation into the aggressive aspects of narcissism', *International Journal of Psycho-Analysis*, 52: 169-78.

Sandler, J. (1976) 'Countertransference and role-responsivenesss', *International Review of Psycho-Analysis*, 3: 43-7.

Segal H. (1950) 'Some aspects of the analysis of a schizophrenic', *International Journal of Psycho-Analysis*, 31: 268-78. Repr. in (1981) *The Work of Hanna Segal* (with a postcript, 1980). New York: Jason Aronson.

—— (1952) 'A psycho-analytical approach to aesthetics', *International journal of Psycho-Analysis*, 33: 96-297. Repr. in (1981) *The Work of Hanna Segal* (with a postcript, 1980). New York: Jason Aronson.

—— (1956) 'Depression in the schizophrenic', *International Journal of Psycho-Analysis*, 37: 339-43. Repr. in (1981) *The Work of Hanna Segal* (with a postcript, 1980). New York: Jason Aronson.

—— (1957) 'Notes on symbol formtion', *International Journal of Psycho-Analysis*, 38: 391-7. Repr. in (1981) *The Work of Hanna Segal* (with a postscript, 1980). New York: Jason Aronson.

—— (1962) 'The curative factors in psychoanalysis', *International Journal of Psychoanalysis*, 43: 212-7. Repr. in (1981) The Work of Hanna Segal (with a postscript, 1980) New York, Jason Aronson.

—— (1964) Introduction to *The Work of Melanie Klein*. London: The Hogarth Press.

—— (1978) 'On symbolism', *International Journal of Psycho-Analysis*, 55: 393-401. Repr. in (1997) *Psychoanalysis, Literature and War*. London: Routledge.

—— (1980) Postscript to 'Schizoid Mechanisms Underlying Phobia Formation' in (1981) *The Work of Hanna Segal*. New York: Jason Aronson.

—— (1981) ' The Function of Dreams' in (1981) *The Work of Hanna Segal*. New York: Jason Aronson.

—— (1984) 'Joseph Conrad and the mid-life crisis', *International Review of Psycho-Analysis*, 11: 3-9. Repr. in (1997) *Psychoanalysis, Literature and War*. London: Routledge.

—— (1987) 'Silence is the real crime', *International Review of Psycho-Analysis*, 14: 3-12. Repr. in (1997) *Psychoanalysis, Literature and War*. London: Routledge.

—— (1989) Introduction to Britton, R. *et al.* eds, *The Oedipus Complex Today*. London: Karnac.

—— (1991) *Dream, Phantasy and Art*, London Routledge

—— (1994) 'Phantasy and reality', *International Journal of Psycho-Analysis*, 75: 359-401. Repr. in (1997) *Psychoanalysis, Literature and War*. London: Routledge.

—— (1995) 'Hiroshima, the Gulf War, and after', in Elliott, A. and Frosh, S. eds, *Psychoanalysis in Contexts: Paths between Theory and Modern Culture*. London: Routledge.

—— (1997) 'The Oedipus Complex Today' in *Psychoanalysis, Literature and War*. London: Routledge.

Steiner, J. (1997) Introduction to *Psychoanalysis, Literature and War*. London: Routledge.

Strachey, J. (1934) 'The nature of the therapeutic action of psychoanalysis', *International journal of Psycho-Analysis*, 15: 127-159. Repr. in *International Journal of Psycho-Analysis* 50: 275-92.

Wollheim R. (1969) 'The mind and the mind's image of itself', *International Journal of Psycho-Analysis* 50: 209-220. Repr. in (1973) Wollheim, *On Art and the Mind*. London: Allen Lane.

1

Symbol Formation and Creativity

Hanna Segal's Theoretical Contributions

Robert Caper, M.D.

Symbol Formation and 'Optimal Anxiety'

Melanie Klein's paper on 'The Importance of Symbol Formation in the Development of the Ego', published in 1930, was a milestone in two respects: first, it opened up the study of symbolisation as a creative and developmental process, and second, it showed how abnormalities in the ability to form symbols could cripple the development of the ego.

Klein suggested that the ego's attachment to its first, few primal objects grows to encompass the wider world only through the development of symbolic links: our interest in the world develops only if new objects can be made to represent our old ones symbolically. Her paper was also of great importance in a third way: it provided the basis for Hanna Segal's work on symbol formation.

It therefore seems appropriate to begin my review of Segal's work with a summary of Klein's paper, which contains an account of her analysis of a four-year old autistic boy, Dick, whose arrested ego development was connected to an almost complete inability to form symbols. Klein's theoretical understanding of this disability was as follows: the young infant is not able to repress its sadism, as it is later on, but expels it into a good object – the mother's body – which it then feels it has destroyed. It experiences this sadism not as a fantasy or wish, but concretely as biting, tearing, stamping, burning, drowning and shooting of the object. At the same time, 'the weapons used to destroy the object are felt by the [infant] to be levelled at his own self as well'.[1]

Klein believed that the anxiety that one felt with regard to the original object (the mother's body) as a result of this projected sadism was an important developmental force, since it propelled the ego away

37

from its exclusive relationship with the original objects toward new objects, which it would then use to represent the older ones symbolically. She placed great emphasis on the importance of symbolic links for normal development because she believed that all contact with internal and external reality was a symbolic displacement of the contact with one's primal objects. In this vein, she wrote that, 'not only does symbolism come to be the foundation of all phantasy and all sublimation, but, more than that, it is the basis of the subject's relation to the outside world and to reality in general' (Klein, 1930, pp. 220-1).

If the child's relationship to reality is to develop in an optimal way, this 'beneficial' anxiety about the original object must be present. But if it is too great, as in Dick's case, rather than propelling one away from the primal object into symbolic relations with new objects, it will paralyse his capacity to form a symbolic relationship with anything. In her discussion of Dick's autism, Klein wrote that

> ... what brought symbol-formation to a standstill was the dread of what would be done to him ... after he had penetrated into his mother's body [in his primitive oedipal phantasies] ... the defence against the sadistic impulse directed against the mother's body and its contents – impulses connected with phantasies of coitus – had resulted in the cessation of phantasies and the standstill of symbol-formation. Dick's further development came to grief because he could not bring into phantasy the sadistic relationship to the mother's body. (Klein, 1930, p. 224)

Symbolic Equation and Confusion of Self and Object

When Klein says that 'Dick's further development came to grief because he could not bring into phantasy the sadistic relationship to the mother's body', she seems to mean that Dick was so frightened of his aggressive impulses that he turned off his phantasising (or at least his aggressive phantasising and impulses) altogether, as a defensive manoeuvre. This left him lacking in the aggression necessary to make his way in the world. But the idea that Dick 'could not bring into phantasy' his sadistic impulses also has other implications: Dick's sadistic impulses, if not brought into fantasy, were left as concrete experiences.

Hanna Segal takes up this point in her first paper on symbol formation, written in 1957. She pointed out that if one's relationship to the external world – one's objects – is extremely concrete (as Dick's was), one will not experience one's thoughts and fantasies about one's objects as thoughts and fantasies, but as concrete actions that one is performing on the actual objects. Segal agreed with Klein that Dick's ability to form

38

symbolic relationships was crippled by overwhelming anxiety about his object (or rather, about his phantasies about it), but added that part of the reason Dick's phantasies were frightening was that Dick did not know that his phantasies were just phantasies; he felt that they were real, concrete acts.

This situation was the product of a state of mind in which Dick had almost completely obliterated the distinction between himself and his object, and this state of mind was in turn produced by the fantasy that he and his objects had concretely entered each other, and lived inside each other. The distinction between himself and his objects having been eliminated in this way, he was unable to distinguish between something that was himself (his fantasies about his objects) and what was in fact not himself (his actual objects).

Segal points out that true symbolisation is a three-part relationship between the thing symbolised, the thing functioning as a symbol, and the person for whom the latter represents the former.

There was something about the quality of Dick's projections into his objects – his 'concrete evacuations of sadism' – that abolished the distinction between himself (or his sadism) and his object. Segal says that the psychotic's projections have this quality because they are not true projections, but projective identifications instead. The 'identification' in projective identification means that the self and object are literally experienced as the same thing. Loss of the self/object distinction leads in turn to loss of his capacity to phantasise and symbolise: if the distinction between two of the three terms (self/object) of the triangular relationship (self/object/symbol) necessary for phantasy and symbol-formation to occur is lost, so is the ability to form true symbols.

This perspective on the psychotic's inability to have an ordinary phantasy life seems to me to be much more interesting and psychological than the one that Klein proposed. Klein, we recall, seems to say that Dick was so terrified of the sadism that he had projected into his mother that he stopped phantasising. But there is something unsatisfactory about this formulation. How does one stop phantasising? Just try it.

Segal proposed that the psychotic does not stop phantasising, but rather develops a phantasy about his phantasies: he believes that his phantasies about his object are literally and concretely true of the object. This is equivalent to confusion between one's phantasies about the object and the object itself. This type of phantasy is no longer a phantasy in the proper sense, but something else instead; Dick could not bring his impulses into phantasy because he was bringing them into this concrete form that is very different from a phantasy in the ordinary sense of the word.[2] Since one's symbols are phantasies, confusion between one's phantasies about one's object and the object itself implies confusion between one's symbols and what they stand for.

Segal proposed that this confused, concrete type of relationship between the symbol and what is symbolised be called a 'symbolic equation'. According to Segal, while symbolic equations are a kind of substitute for the original objects, 'they are hardly different from the original object. These substitutes are treated as though they were *identical* with it ... The symbolic equation between the original object and the symbol in the internal and external world is, I think, the basis of the schizophrenic's concrete thinking'.

The distinction between a symbol and a symbolic equation, like that between the depressive and paranoid-schizoid positions, is schematic. In fact, during normal development there is a gradual transition from a state of mind dominated by symbolic equations and one dominated by symbolisation proper. This transition stems from the growing ability to acknowledge that the good object is not oneself. This is sometimes referred to as the loss (or renunciation) of the object; this does not refer to an actual external loss, but rather to an inner acknowledgement that the object is not the self.

This acknowledgement permits the use of symbols in a less concrete way. Segal (1957) points out that this in turn has two important psychological consequences. First,

> The capacity to experience loss and the wish to re-create the object within oneself gives the individual the unconscious freedom in the use of symbols. And as the symbol is acknowledged as a creation of the subject, unlike the symbolic equation, it can be used freely by the subject.

This means that one has acquired the capacity to use one's symbols and phantasies in a free, imaginative way.

The second point has to do with the ego's ever-widening use of new objects as symbolic representations of old ones:

> When a substitute in the external world is used as a symbol, it may be used more freely than the original object, since it is not fully identified with it. But inasmuch as it is distinguished from the original object, the symbol is also recognised as an object in itself. Its own properties are recognised, respected and used because no confusion with the original object blurs the characteristics of the new object used as a symbol.

40

1. Symbol Formation and Creativity

This means that one has also acquired the capacity to see new objects and new experiences as they really are – distinct from one's phantasies about them or symbolic use of them. For example, the Earth may be a symbol for the mother, but only by being able to see how the earth *differs* from a mother can one acquire geological knowledge – knowledge of the earth as it really is. By the same token, if we recognise that the Earth is not really mother, but only a symbol for her (as, indeed, the word 'mother' is), we can be free to use it for our creative purposes in ways that we could never use our actual mothers.

Segal's work indicates that imaginativeness, on the one hand, and a realistic outlook – the ability to see the world as it actually is – on the other, far from being opposed to each other (as in the false antithesis between the creative artist and the scientist), are both products of the same psychological accomplishment.

A third important contribution contained in this paper is Segal's insight into the role that symbol formation plays in normal repression (which differs from splitting or projection in that one has greater contact with what has been repressed than with what has been split off):

> Symbols are needed not only in communication with the external world, but also in internal communication. Indeed, it could be asked what is meant when we speak of people being in touch with the unconscious. It is not that they have consciously primitive phantasies, like those which become evident in their analyses, but merely that they have some awareness of their own impulses and feelings. However, I think that we mean more than this; we mean they have an actual *communication* with their unconscious phantasies. And this, like any other form of communication can be done only with the help of symbols. So that in people who are 'in touch with themselves' there is a constant free symbol formation, whereby they can be consciously aware and in control of *symbolic expressions* of the underlying primitive phantasies. The difficulty in dealing with schizophrenic and schizoid patients lies not only in their failure to communicate with us but even more in their failure to communicate with themselves.

The availability of lines of symbolic communication between the conscious and the unconscious in normal subjects, and the lack of it in schizophrenic and schizoid states of mind, is one of the crucial differences between normal repression and splitting.

At this point, Segal's work on symbolisation makes contact with Bion's theory of thinking. We may compare the idea of 'being in touch with oneself' as symbolic communication with the unconscious with

Bion's notion of the contact-barrier that separates the normal conscious mind from the normal unconscious mind in normal repression.

Bion pictured this barrier as a kind of network or mesh work composed of what he called alpha-elements. These elements are like true symbols in the sense that they represent some aspect of reality, but are still recognised as being separate from what they represent. Alpha-elements may be contrasted with beta-elements in Bion's model, since beta-elements are experienced as identical with what they represent (as 'things-in-themselves'). In this regard, the difference between an alpha and a beta-element is the same as the difference between a symbol and a symbolic equation.

In Bion's model, a barrier composed of alpha-elements allows contact between our conscious and unconscious minds. This contact is symbolic: the alpha-elements are symbols of what is unconscious or repressed. But the contact-barrier also keeps the conscious and unconscious separate, because there is still the recognition that these symbols are just symbols and not the contents of the unconscious itself.

Symbolism and Projective Identification

Segal's next important contribution to the theory of symbol formation, 'On symbolism' (Segal, 1978), appeared as part of a colloquium on symbol formation at the International Psychoanalytic Congress in Jerusalem in 1977. It begins with a summary of some of the points of her 1957 paper, followed by a revision of her 1957 view that projective identification *per se* leads to concretisation and symbolic equations. She now says that this is an oversimplification: the nature of the projective identification and its fate in the object also have to be taken into account. This modification of her views seems to be in response to Bion's extension of the concept of projective identification to include 'normal projective identification' alongside the type described originally by Klein, which is now qualified as excessive or pathological projective identification.

Projective Identification into Reality

Segal illustrates what she means by the fate of the projective identification with a clinical example of a man who had an extremely vivid and frightening dream, almost indistinguishable from a hallucination, of a motorcyclist riding into his forehead. Now, the patient was prone to fantasies of intruding on and invading the analyst (representing his mother), and the details of the dream and his associations to it showed that such fantasies of intrusive projective identification into the mother/analyst played a part in its formation. That is, his phantasies of intruding upon or invading the analyst made him experience the analyst as invading him in the form of a motorcycle.

But the dream was also connected to the previous session which had in fact been intruded upon by the noise from motorcycles just outside the consulting room window. The patient connected motorcycles with the analyst's son. This actual intrusion repeated a childhood situation in which a very intrusive older brother interfered with the patient's relationship to his mother even when he was a tiny baby. So the 'fate' of this particular projective identification was to encounter a reality, both in the patient's past and in the present, which was congruent with it, and this contributed to making the experience and the dream so concrete.

The point here is that the reality into which one is projecting must also be taken into account, since if the reality is too similar to that which is projected into it, one may experience one's phantasies in a concrete way that will interfere with symbol formation and abstract thought.[3]

Destructive Projective Identification

Segal's next point is that the nature of the projective identification itself must be taken into account:

A great deal of work has been done on projective identification since Melanie Klein formulated it, particularly by Bion in his work on the relation between the containing and the contained and Herbert Rosenfeld in his work on narcissism. The fate of development in the depressive position is largely determined by the vicissitudes of projective identification. Bion's (1957) model, which I find the most helpful, is as follows. The child projects into the breast unbearable feelings. The mother elaborates them, and if she gives an appropriate response, the child can introject the breast as a container capable of dealing with feelings. The introjection of such a container is the necessary precondition for the elaboration of the depressive position. But a great deal can go wrong with the projection. The relationship between the container and contained may be felt as mutually destructive or mutually emptying, as well as being mutually creative. If the relationship between the container and contained is of a positive nature, the depressive elaboration and the depressive symbol formation can proceed. If the relationship is disturbed, it immediately affects the nature of the symbol formation (p. 317).

43

She then presents material from a second patient, illustrating how the nature of the projective identification itself may lead to a bad relationship between the container and the contained, producing 'extreme difficulty in communicating'.

At times, this patient responded to interpretation with physical sensations; she felt that the analyst's words were concrete things. These were times when she felt that her projections had totally and concretely identified themselves with the container – that she had invaded the analyst's mind and made it into her physical possession.

At other times, her speech became highly abstract, technical and full of jargon and clichés – in other words, devoid of meaning. Simultaneously, she emptied the analyst's words of meaning by immediately translating them into some philosophical or psychoanalytical abstract term or concept. She also felt empty of meaning herself – she didn't know, or couldn't say, what she meant. At these times, container and contained have a mutually emptying type of relationship.

The mutually destructive relationship between container and contained was related to this patient's envy and narcissism, as a result of which 'nothing is allowed to exist outside herself that could give rise to envy'.[4]

Containment and Meaningful Speech

In my opinion, Segal's most original contribution in this paper concerns her use of Bion's theory of the container as a model for the acquisition of meaningful speech. 'The infant', she writes, 'has had an experience and mother provides a word or phrase which circumscribes the experience. It contains, encompasses and expresses the meaning. It provides a container for it. The infant can then internalise the word or phrase containing the meaning'.

In addition to being a model of some aspects of the acquisition of meaningful speech, this is a very good model of an important facet of the psychoanalytic process. In analysis, it is the analyst's job to find the appropriate word – the word that contains, encompasses and expresses the meaning of the patient's unconscious experience. Recall that Freud held that the only way for an unconscious idea to become conscious was for it to become attached to a word. While today we may not put as much emphasis on verbal representation and verbal symbols as Freud did,[5] doing analysis is largely a mater of finding the right words. We may paint pictures with our interpretations, but they are word pictures.

Once the analyst has circumscribed the patient's experience with a word,[6] the patient can internalise the word or interpretation containing the experience. This means not only that the interpretation must encompass the unconscious experience adequately – be worthy of internalising – but also that the patient be able to experience the value of the interpretation so that he wants to take it inside himself – in other words, to recognise that the interpretation is worth internalising.

Segal's second patient had the greatest difficulty experiencing any interpretation as containing and giving expression to meaning, and hence as being worth internalising. An important root of this difficulty came to light when she reported a dream in which she was a little girl with long nails and ferocious teeth greedily attacking a table, scratching and biting. She associated this to having read a book about a little girl who lost her sight and hearing and was like a wild little animal until the day she invented a sign language and taught it to her teacher.

The book was Helen Keller's autobiography, but the patient had turned one crucial detail completely around. In the actual autobiography, for a long time Helen's '... teacher had tried to communicate with her by writing on her hand. Helen did not respond. After a long period of breaking and smashing and unconcern, one day she broke a doll and, for the first time, cried. That afternoon when the teacher tried again to communicate with her and wrote a word on her palm, Helen Keller understood and responded. Thus, a capacity to understand symbolic communication followed immediately and directly from that first experience of depressive feelings'.

Segal's patient had still to accept that she learned to speak from her parents, but she was prevented from doing this by her narcissism and envy, which forced her to claim that it was the other way around.

Symbol Formation and Creativity

Segal's work on the disorders of symbol formation has lead to a greater understanding of the creative use of symbols as well. In her paper on 'Delusion and artistic creativity' (Segal, 1974), she uses the material of William Golding's novel *The Spire* to investigate the nature of creativity. This is a fascinating paper that I cannot hope to summarise here, but I would like to mention one aspect of it, since it bears directly on her work on symbol formation. The novel takes place in the middle ages and its protagonist, Jocelin, is the dean of a cathedral who dreams of adding to it a 400 foot spire. He claims that the spire will reflect the glory of God, but it is clear from the story that it is his own glory that he wishes it to reflect (he plans to have his own image on all four sides of the spire, and he compares the completed structure to a man's body, with the gigantic spire arising from the middle).

Jocelin cannot built his spire without the aid of a master builder, Roger Mason, who refuses to co-operate because he does not believe that the structure will stand; the cathedral's foundations are too weak to support it. Excavation proves the builder right, but this only strengthens Jocelin's determination to proceed.

The contrast between Jocelin and Roger Mason is one between grandiose, delusional narcissism and sober realism. But it is also a contrast between sterility and creativity. Jocelin claims that the spire is an expression of love for his object – God – but it is clear that he has identified himself with God and that the spire is really an expression of his love for an idealised image of himself. He is incapable of constructing anything real, however, because he sacrifices his perception of reality for the sake of maintaining his narcissistic delusions. Like the cathedral, his delusional system lacks foundation in reality. Roger Mason's view of what he can do is constrained by reality, and is hence much more modest, but, unlike Jocelin, he is capable of creating something real.

One of the points I believe Segal is making in this paper is that, for our symbolic work to be creative, it must symbolise something real. She makes a similar point in a different way in her paper on 'A psychoanalytic approach to aesthetics' (Segal, 1952), in which she describes a case of a young girl

> … with a definite gift for painting. An acute rivalry with her mother had made her give up painting in her early teens. After some analysis she started to paint again and was working as a decorative artist. She did decorative handicraft work in preference to what she sometimes called 'real painting', and this was because she knew that, though correct, neat and pretty, her work failed to be moving and aesthetically significant. In her manic way, she usually denied that this caused her any concern. At the time when I was trying to interpret her unconscious sadistic attacks on her father, the internalisation of her mutilated and destroyed father, and the resulting depression, she told me the following dream: She had seen a picture in a shop which represented a wounded man lying alone and desolate in a dark forest. She felt quite overwhelmed with emotion and admiration for this picture; she thought it represented the actual essence of life; if she could only paint like that she would be a really great painter.
>
> It soon appeared that the meaning of the dream was that if she could only acknowledge her depression about the wounding and destruction of her father, she would then be able to express it in her painting and would

achieve real art ... her dream showed something that had not been in any way indicated or interpreted by me: namely the effect on her painting of her persistent denial of depression.

The patient's creativity had been stifled by her refusal to acknowledge reality, in this case the reality of her inner world. Only if, like the builder in Golding's novel, she could allow herself to be *constrained* by reality could she accomplish something substantial – 'be a really great painter'. While it is quite obvious that someone working in the practical world must pay attention to reality – an architect or builder must obey the laws of physics or his creation will literally come crashing down around his ears – Segal is making the point here that the same thing is true for other forms of creativity as well.

I believe that this is an important point about creativity that deserves greater emphasis than it usually receives. Our symbolic creations must symbolise things as they are, which means we must accept that what we are symbolising is not of our own making (even though our symbols are) and that the significance and value of our symbolic creations depends on their being constrained by the reality that they represent. Joshua Reynolds wrote that

> on the whole, it seems to me that there is but one presiding principle which regulates what gives stability to every art. The works, whether of poets, painters, moralists or historians, which are built upon general nature, live forever; while those which depend for their existence on particular customs and habits, a partial view of nature, or the fluctuations of fashion can only be coeval with that which first raised them from obscurity.

A symbol must be true to what is real, including the reality of our inner world. This is the difference between a symbol, which is subordinate to what it symbolises, and a symbolic equation, which takes over and replaces what it is supposed to represent, as Jocelin's spire did with God.

When artistic creativity is viewed in this light, one becomes hard pressed to distinguish purely artistic creations from scientific creativity. Both true artistic creations and creative scientific theories owe their validity to their being faithfully subservient to some reality beyond the investigator's control.

Symbol Formation and the Oedipal Situation

I would like to conclude with a point that Segal made recently about the practice of psychoanalysis that is connected to her work on symbol formation. In a 'Dialogue on Countertransference' held at the International Psychoanalytic Congress in 1993, she suggested that the analyst must have the capacity to be affected by the patient's projections – to form countertransference – in order to be sensitive to the patient. But, she added, he must also be able to distance himself from the projection so he may *observe* the countertransference.

The patient experiences this distance as the analyst having a relationship with something or someone other than the patient. Segal suggests that this is a realistic perception. The analyst, she said, is indeed in a triangular relationship with the patient, on the one hand, and his internal objects, on the other. My own experience confirms this: the so-called analytic dyad is actually a triad, and the analyst must be able to maintain at least two relationships at once – with his patient and with his internal objects – if he is to be able to analyse the patient's projected communications.

Absorbing a patient's projections so they may generate a countertransference in the analyst, while at the same time maintaining a critical distance from it so it may be recognised as a countertransference resulting from the patient's projections, is a very difficult ask. But recognition of one's countertransference and through that the nature and function of the patient's projections seems to be an essential part of doing psychoanalysis.

I believe that there is a special internal object that helps the analyst to do analysis. The object is psychoanalysis itself, as a source of a particular kind of truth, and it is an *internal* object if the analyst loves psychoanalysis and the truths it brings. His devotion to the internal object allows him to be in contact with the patient's projections, while protecting him from over-identifying with them. It is acquired and strengthened through the analyst's own analysis, and its presence seems to be a good criterion of that elusive state called 'being analysed', or 'having an identity as a psychoanalyst'.

The analyst's relationship with this internal object is like the mother's relationship with the father that allows her to be in contact with the baby, while protecting her from becoming fused with or dominated by it. If the analyst behaves like a mother in being receptive to the patient's projections, in distancing himself from them he is acting like a father that comes between the infant and mother. In doing both at the same time, that is, in doing psychoanalysis, he is acting like a parental couple.

This triangular relationship between the receptive analyst, the patient, and something in the analyst that keeps the patient from dominating and possessing him, is a real oedipal situation. Segal said that when the patient becomes aware of the analyst's relationship with this internal object, which keeps him from being able to dominate the analyst with his projections, he may be filled with hatred. We are used to interpreting our patient's reaction to breaks in the analysis in terms of oedipal conflicts. But could it be that the analyst's capacity to interpret the patient's projections, which gives evidence of his link to an internal analytic object is an even more powerful oedipal experience than analytic breaks, since it gives the patient direct and immediate evidence that the analyst is having a relationship with someone else?

If, as I am suggesting, the interpretation itself places the patient in an oedipal relationship with the analyst, then the patient's relationship to the interpretation – his capacity to allow the analyst to make the interpretation, to take it in and to preserve it in his mind – depends in part on the degree to which he is able to work through the oedipal situation with which the interpretation itself presents him.

In addition to this, if we consider what it means to be in contact with one's feelings, wishes, fantasies and perceptions, we realise that it implies being receptive to them (that is, not denying them, splitting them off or projecting them), while at the same time keeping a certain distance from them, so that we experience them merely as our fantasies or feelings, and not as concrete realities. In other words, we are in contact with them without being dominated by them. This relationship with our own minds is the same as the analyst's relationship to the patient's mind. I do not believe that this is merely coincidental; the state of mind that enables the patient to use an interpretation is the same as the one that allows him to be in symbolic contact with himself.

Clinical Illustration

I would like to illustrate these points with an excerpt from the analysis of a young woman who, at the time of her analysis, was working toward a degree in ancient history. One of her major symptoms was an inhibition of self-expression. This symptom was connected to a fear that her ideas would not harmonise with the listener's, and that the listener would then attack her because of the difference. At times, this inhibition led her to become confused about what her ideas really were.

She began a Monday session by saying that she had spent the weekend attending a seminar in her field. It was 'OK', she said, but she found that she had got into an unpleasant, 'spaced-out' state of mind that she could not bring herself out of. All she could say about the weekend was that she felt that one of her professors was too solicitous of everyone, and that this 'drove her crazy', for reasons that she was unable to put into words. This state of mind was familiar from previous work in the analysis. It usually meant that she had lost contact with her inner world – her thoughts and emotions. But beyond this general assessment, nothing emerged.

In the following session, however, she reported a dream in which

> she was about to have sexual intercourse with a man she loves when she noticed that there was a baby in the room. It seemed to be about one and a half or two years old – she wasn't sure. In any event, just as her lover was about to penetrate her, she found she could not let him with the child in the room. The dream repeats, this time with her turned away from the child, but the same thing happens again: the child's presence plays on her mind and stops her love-making.

In the third session of the week, she reported that she found herself 'spacing out' again the previous night, as she had during her weekend seminar. This occurred while she had been talking to a friend about a historian whose views on Athenian democracy she consciously believed she shared. She began to feel bored, and this led to the spaced-out feeling of detachment from herself. She said this was odd, because she had always been interested in the ideas that this author discusses. She had felt detached from herself since then. Her interest in the author's work was based on a feeling that his ideas led naturally to certain ideas of her own about the paradoxical coexistence of democracy and slavery in ancient Athens. The problem of an aristocratic slave-based system existing within a democracy was important to her because she felt it had practical implications for the race problem in the United States. In fact, she had recently thought of someday writing something that would bring the author's ideas together with hers – to show the harmony between them.

But what emerged after some discussion (and considerable resistance) was that she was denying that the author was working very hard *not* to talk about the ideas that are so important to her, even when they appeared to follow from what he is saying – that he is actually hostile to them. This surprised her greatly, but she realised it must be true, and after some reflection she said that she thought she was trying to eliminate some important differences between herself and the author, to avoid the possibility of conflict between herself and him because she admired much of what he had to say. She then realised that this is what annoyed her about her professor over the weekend – he wanted everyone at the seminar to be one big happy family, but in a crazy way. He seemed to feel responsible for bringing everyone into harmony and making them all comfortable with each other's views. The link between the weekend situation and the dream was now evident: in the dream her intercourse was stopped by her fear that it would cause a disharmonious relationship with the child. She was unable to let herself feel real passion for someone she loved because that would disrupt the requirement that she create one big family that brought the sexual couple together with the left-out child in a completely harmonious way, free of jealousy and envy.

In retrospect, we may see that in her dream, she was doing what her professor had done over the weekend, and that she was driven by a need to maintain harmony, as she felt her professor was. But why was it *she* in the dream and not her professor (that is, why was she identified with her professor) and why did the dream portray the family situation in oedipal terms? I believe that these questions may be partly answered by reviewing some other aspects of the patient's analysis.

This patient often resists interpretations in a way that is quite subtle and difficult to detect. While appearing to agree with them, she will bend their meaning slightly so that they harmonise with what she is already conscious of. She does this in such a way that the revised interpretation sounds reasonable, but only in a superficial way. On other occasions, she will quibble about some peripheral part of the interpretation, so that the main point – the point that had disturbed her – gets lost. This too creates a spurious 'harmony' between her ideas and mine. The effect of the manoeuvre is to leave me confused about what I had meant in the first place – out of touch with myself.

The reason that she appeared in the dream instead of her professor was that what 'drove her crazy' was not only an aspect of his personality, but of hers as well. It was this aspect of her own personality, projected into her professor, that drove her crazy over the weekend. In forming her dream, she had projected this aspect of herself once again, but this time into the baby. In the dream, she feels that the baby would be disturbed by witnessing adult sexuality, and this disturbs her to the point that she is unable to consummate the act. She is disturbed by the baby's disturbance because it is really an aspect of herself – one that insists on harmony at all costs, even if it means eliminating the differences between babies and adults.

The question of why this dream was sexual requires a more complex answer. This patient is very grateful when she feels that I have been able to make an interpretation with enough conviction to prevent her from 'harmonising' it into something less disturbing. My conviction arises, I believe, from my being able to establish a clear enough contact with my unconscious as it is affected by her unconscious projections and communications. This is *not* precisely the same as contact with her, and this is a critical point. It is contact with an aspect of myself that enables me to make proper analytic contact with her unconscious. The confusion that she projects as part of her resistance is an attempt to interrupt the contact with my unconscious that I rely on to make proper analytic contact with her. She is unconsciously aware that my ability to analyse her depends on my being in contact with my unconscious, and that this contact excludes her (even as it helps me to recognise what she is unconsciously projecting and communicating); it is private.

The situation I am trying to describe is represented perfectly by picturing the analyst as a parental *couple*, a mother receiving the infant's (patient's) projections, but who is also in relation to a father, who prevents the projections from taking the receptive mother over. That is, the baby is able to *communicate* to the mother, but is not able to get inside her and consume her with its projections. The reason for this is that the sexual father is already inside the mother; he has preempted that position. To say the same thing in different terms, it is the mother's love for the father that establishes him as an internal object for her. Her love for the baby allows her to be receptive to it, and her love for the father protects her from being dominated by the baby. This accounts for the sexual character of the dream. The conflict the patient experiences when I make an interpretation arises from an aspect of herself, represented by the baby, that interferes with my internal analytic intercourse with myself. It also, through identification with the split-up couple, interferes with her being able to establish a similar contact with herself – to know clearly what she thinks – and with her being able to have a good analytic intercourse with me. The dream was over determined, and represented all three aspects of her conflict.

This interpretation of the dream is supported by the next (Thursday) session, which she began by saying that she felt much better after the Wednesday session. She now found herself feeling quite angry with the author. She couldn't believe she felt that strongly 'about a book'. She then related a dream in which she was given a box by an old friend whose face had always 'looked much younger than his age'. He warned her that the box contained scorpions, but when she accidentally dropped it, she found that it was actually full of harmless spiders instead. The sight of them crawling all over the carpet 'made her itch'. She tried to blow them into a corner in an attempt to gather them back into the box, but without success. Then someone said they were dangerous and must be burned. There was a fiery explosion and she ran away, fearing that her night-gown, flowing behind her, had caught fire and that she would burn. She associated the spiders to the family gathering of the previous weekend, where two or three babies were crawling on the carpet. She was distressed when she realised that the babies' mothers were ignoring them.

In this dream, the baby-faced friend represents an omnipotent baby that presents itself as a powerful and dangerous scorpion (i.e., that she *feels* is a powerful and dangerous scorpion). When she realises that it is really a harmless crawler, associated to a neglected baby, she tries to put it back in its place. But there is an explosion apparently connected to a resurgence of the feeling that the baby is dangerous. The resulting fire threatens to burn her night-gown, and her along with it.

The scorpion's sting is the pang of guilt that my patient felt in the first dream over exposing the baby to adult sexuality. The guilt is based on the idea that she and her objects should all be one big happy family – that they should be unaware of any real difference between them that might give rise to envy or jealousy. When she recognised in the Wednesday session how destructive this idea can be to her contact with herself, she was able to overcome the guilt, and the scorpion once more became just a left-out, harmless spider-baby. But the baby, as if enraged by her progress in detaching herself from it, then counterattacks with a fire storm, a form of attack that is more overtly directed against her sexuality (the night-gown).

The scorpion/arsonist represented an aspect of herself that was furious with her parents' sexuality, and that she felt was able to put a stop to it. But since my patient was not conscious of ever having felt jealous of her parents' sexual relationship (since she never believed there was much to be jealous about), my interpretation about the scorpion and the incendiary representing an oedipal aspect of herself left her interested, but unmoved. A few weeks later, however, she had another dream in which

she saw her mother emerge from a room, shirtless, with a man who placed his hand on her bare breast. The patient 'got hysterical and threw a fit', yelling and screaming at her mother for 'betraying her father'. Later in the dream, she tells her father of the betrayal, but he seems oddly philosophical about it. His *sang-froid* raised the suspicion that the man with whom her mother committed her act of betrayal was the father himself (disguised as someone else in line with her denial that her parents were ever passionate with each other) and the betrayal over which she became so upset was a betrayal of the patient herself: her mother's feeding breast becoming a sexual breast. This accords with the ferocity of her reaction, which was what impressed the patient most of all about the dream. She had not recalled ever having such strong feelings about her mother. In this last dream, *she* is now the baby in the first dream: the projection of her jealousy and envy has been reversed, and she is now in better contact with herself.

When I was able in the analysis to make interpretations based on my internal analytic function, and at the same time withstand her attempts to undermine it, I represented to her a combined parental figure – a mother who is in contact with the baby, and also a father who prevents the baby from making contact with the mother in a destructive way by invading her relationship with the father to form a 'happy' family. The first dream represents not only her attempts to make contact with herself, but also this situation in the analysis, where she is the oedipal baby witnessing my intercourse with my internal analytic object. The two parallel meanings of this dream indicate the close relationship between the ability to allow the analyst to make interpretations – to allow the parents to be a sexual couple – and to think for oneself – to allow an intercourse to occur between different aspects of one's personality. The former reflects an acceptance that one's objects have lives of their own, and passionate relationships with one another that one can only observe without being part of or controlling. The latter reflects an acceptance that one's mind has a life if its own, and passions that one can only observe and know about without controlling. If we can accept this, then we can know what we think and feel in a connected yet separate way: that is, we are able to think symbolically.

Conclusion

Klein observed that it was Dick's Oedipal relationship with his mother – the realisation that she contained within herself a relationship with his father – that most filled him with the hatred and sadism that crippled his ability to think symbolically. My examination of Segal's enrichment and broadening of Klein's work on symbol-formation has come around full circle to return to Klein's insight that the capacity to think symbolically is a consequence of having accepted one's position in the family *vis à vis* one's parents. Perhaps we might also say that one's very sanity – the acknowledgement of one's true position in the world – is itself an expression of one's acceptance of these primary oedipal realities, and that one of the pre-conditions for a truly creative state of mind may be sanity in this sense.

Notes

1. In this regard, the sadism that Klein describes is similar to destructive narcissism (Rosenfeld, 1971), which attacks both the good object and the healthy dependent self.

2. One could add that the phenomena that Segal delineated in this paper written 35 years ago belong, to the domain of what we would now call narcissistic object relationships. The paralysing anxiety over what one feels the object contains, alluded to by Klein, and the confusion between self and object that Segal emphasised are both manifestations of narcissistic hatred of the good object separate from the self. This hatred causes one to attack the object and to confuse oneself with it, doing both in an attempt to eliminate one's perception of what one hates: an object that is both good and separate from the self. The result is a bad, attacking object that one cannot escape and is even hopelessly confused with.

3. This insight provides an important clue about the mechanism of action of pathogenic environments. For example, in cases of actual incest, the close correspondence between the reality and the child's oedipal phantasies may cause the child later in life to experience its sexual phantasies in a concrete, non-symbolic way. How much of the psychopathology of the incest victim may be accounted for in this way?

4. This is, of course, a description of narcissistic hatred of the good object referred to above.

5. Non-verbal images can also serve quite well as symbols of unconscious content, and do so not infrequently in dreams. Music is also capable of encompassing and evoking quite complex emotional states.

6. 'Word' needs to be taken rather loosely here; it includes complex interpretations, or a series of interpretations, usually re-worked and refined over a considerable period of time to make it a better approximation of the patient's unconscious experience and to tie it in with other interpretations and experiences. This point is illustrated by the fact that a word used in the middle of an analysis may have vastly richer meaning than the same word used at the beginning of an analysis.

References

Klein, M. (1930) 'The Importance of Symbol Formation in the Development of the Ego', in *The Writings of Melanie Klein*, vol. 1: *Love, Guilt and*

Reparation and Other Works, 1921-1945, Hogarth Press, London, (1975), pp. 219-32.

Rosenfeld, H. (1971) 'A clinical approach to the psychoanalytic theory of the life and death instincts: an investigation into the aggressive aspects of narcissism', *International Journal of Psycho-Analysis*, 52: 169-78.

Segal, Hanna (1952) 'A Psychoanalytical Approach to Aesthetics', in *The Work of Hanna Segal*, Jason Aronson, New York, (1981).

—— (1957), 'Notes on symbol formation', *International Journal of Psycho-Analysis*, 38: 391-7. Also in *The Work of Hanna Segal*, Jason Aronson, New York, (1981).

—— (1974) 'Delusion and Artistic Creativity', in *The Work of Hanna Segal*, Jason Aronson, New York, (1981).

—— (1978) 'On symbolism', *International Journal of Psycho-Analysis*, 59: 310-20.

2

Unprovoked Assaults

Making Sense of Apparently Random Violence

Leslie Sohn

The following situation will be termed an unprovoked assault. A totally innocent person is physically attacked, usually in a public place – and not infrequently a very crowded place. The victim has no idea why it has happened to him and the violence of the attack is such that he not infrequently finds himself near death. Yet hitherto the assaulter and the victim have neither met nor known anything about each other.

I have been part of a team in a special forensic unit. Using data derived from three treatments I want to tie together the victim and his attacker in the attacker's mind, setting out to explain how the victim fits the need of a psychotic man's fantasy, at a particular time. In this way an attempt is made to make some sense of an apparently senseless event.

The Treatment Setting

My ideas are based on a series of meetings, in a medium secure hospital, with ten patients.[1] The initial presentation of the three patients whom I am going to describe in detail was a keen wish to speak and to be spoken to, not necessarily about. The first two, PH and ME, could not be said by any means to have been psychoanalysed in my meetings with them; they each had about 150 sessions over a period of about eighteen months. The circumstances of their stay in the unit (which initially was going to be relatively short-term) and the emphasis of the therapeutic approach, was predominantly directed to a curative short-term admission to be followed by out-patient supervision in the community. The psychotherapy with me was in addition to their general psychiatric treatment.

Nonetheless, if I were to have to answer seriously what about these two patients' psychotherapy could not be termed a psychoanalysis, I would be at a loss. The most obvious discrepancies were the duration and the time variations in their sessions and the intentions of the analyst (myself).

The actual sessions were no different from what I undertake in my usual psychoanalytic practice, apart from the fact that they took place in a medium-secure in-patient setting – during which the patients' freedom to move around freely outside was curtailed. Yet even this discrepancy lessened. Towards the end of their sessions with me both patients had almost completely free outside movements.

As far as a difference in my intentions as psychoanalyst is concerned, what I have in mind is that although I maintained an interpretative/analytical posture throughout, I did not intend to be involved with their treatment as out-patients. The treatment was time-limited and this limited my relationship with them.

The setting for the third patient, JP, was quite different. From the outset the very nature of his referral to the Unit allowed for a long-term engagement with this man's treatment. There were no limitations of time – his future was intimately related to long-term treatment – and I was conscious throughout of the fact that should there be any untoward developments in his illness and therefore in his therapy, I could rely on a full back-up system for further in-patient care on the unit. JP was also, from the start, interested in and able to maintain the capacity to be a psychoanalytic patient. In his case, therefore, we met regularly over a three-year period (four times a week) and in this respect the treatment was quite similar to psychoanalysis.

Another essential difference from my ordinary psychoanalytic work was that all three patients received anti-psychotic medication, the control of which lay in the hands of psychiatric colleagues.

Finally, as a further complication to the setting, all three patients were under varying categories of legal compulsion to be where they were. This is in the very nature of their treatment in a medium-secure unit. They had to be clearly told at the onset of their seeing me that they could expect confidentiality but only if there was no breach of security involved in what was concerning us. Our contractual relationship would allow me to notify the Unit authorities if such a breach occurred. Fortunately, this never took place.

2. Unprovoked Assaults

First Patient: PH

PH, aged 33 when I first saw him, was referred from a prison under a specific legal order.[2] Earlier in that same year he had assaulted an elderly man who was a complete stranger.

He had a long history of psychosis, and had been in numerous mental hospitals both in the United Kingdom and abroad. He is one of six children. An elder brother is reported to have committed suicide thirteen years ago, but there is no other official history of mental illness in the family. His early years were spent in the UK and he and the family then moved abroad, the father having an academic post in a research Unit.

His first admission to a mental hospital occurred at the age of 18. A series of admissions followed. The diagnoses then, and in those mental hospitals to which he was admitted on his return to the UK ten years ago, were all confidently of schizophrenia. Anti-psychotic medication was given, and on two occasions he was given antidepressants as well. He seems to have been abandoned by his family – who sent him back to the UK to live with his grandmother. I came to consider this an act of supreme foolhardiness and neglectfulness.

The clinical picture throughout was of auditory hallucinations, grandiose delusional ideas, and restless wanderings. He was living in squats[3] and had short periods in prison. Occasionally he was restless and reported to be sexually uninhibited.

After the attack on the old man, on admission to the unit where I was working, he was thought-disordered. He would change the subject of his thoughts frequently, and there would be no apparent relationship at all between the ideas he expressed. He said there were people out to get him: he alternated between being a member of the SAS (a special commando group) and of the Luftwaffe.

However, as our meetings continued, gradually he was able to talk to me about his very satisfying fantasy mental life. He lives in a fantasy delusional world peopled by famous pop stars, with whom he is on first name terms. Among the pop stars in this fantasy he 'has' a girlfriend and they all live together in complete harmony. In this world the sky is always blue and cloudless. It is a world with no threats. Unfortunately periodically the 'clouds would come over and darken the world'.

He said to me 'You see it would become very dark and threatening. I couldn't get into contact with M (the delusional girlfriend). I found MJ (a pop star) never spoke, I felt heavy and sleepless, I could just about get myself around but no more'. In connection with this he admitted to

59

me that there had been six or seven assaultative events of varying seriousness prior to the one against the old man. He had never been charged with any of them but he knew they had always occurred when the clouds – the really dark clouds – came over.

I came to see that there was an almost compulsive awareness in his behaviour during these phases when he felt troubled by clouds in his inner world. He almost knew quite consciously how he could 'cure' himself: if he would go out into the cloudy world and attack somebody that would make him better. I consider that in this way he knew that he had become depressed but could not tolerate it. Such depressive intrusions into the psychotic world of such a man were totally untenable for him. He needed to project them into somebody by the actual act of violent physical assault. His concrete thinking and rigidity of mind required (a) the act and (b) a resulting conviction that somebody else contained the evil black-clouded experience.

He told me he could remember two of the victims of his attempts to cure himself. The significant thing about them was that they were totally free of any sign of misery – this is his own description of them. He found that he felt them to be totally careless of him and his state of mind. He became convinced that the act of violence towards them freed him and then enveloped them. He reported no feeling of sorrow for his victims' new 'predicament'.

Gradually, I learned more about his early life. His apparent lack of success at school had infuriated his father, who ignored him. He described his mother as 'at his father's service' and quick to be ever available. His grandmother's failure to care for him (which was highly understandable because of his unmanageability) revived, and confirmed, in an absolute way, his experience of a deprived childhood. The real world for him really has been cold and inhospitable.

In the sessions, he constantly referred back to his mother being at the service of his academically successful father. He saw his father as a man in a state of constant satisfaction: mental, physical and sexual. It was as if his parents were in a state of constant sexual activity and satisfaction supplied by his mother's acquiescence and collusion. It seemed quite clear to me that he identified with these copulating parents. The delusional world in which he lived unconsciously repeated the situation he felt should be his. In his mind he could call up M (the girlfriend) as well as MJ (the famous pop star) and feel they would respond to his every wish whenever he wanted.

The essential quality of this onanistic world in which my patient lived was that it was a flow of perfect satisfaction, pleasure and richness. I, therefore, saw the arrival of the black clouds of depression as connected to some occasional recognition of what was felt to be a *loss* of wholly good, albeit idealised and delusional, objects.

A complicating feature here was that he could play an alternating heterosexual and homosexual role in his fantasies. I believe this enabled him to be both the combined parent and to be each at once. Such mental procedures could not improve his mental state or lead to development. Such identifications dissolve the normal knowledge and experience that is required to develop, mature and meet loss and change.

I have found the facts I have now set out concerning PH to be almost routine for such an illness, but they do not explain why getting rid of an experience of this particular form of loss cannot occur psychologically, albeit delusionally, via a projection. To complicate the picture still further, this inhibition of projection was not total. I could observe how, with regularity and efficiency, he could deal with experiences evoking feelings of envy and jealousy – whether it was envy of his father's intellectual or social capabilities and their resultant satisfactions, or jealousy of his parents' relationship as he experienced it. In these cases it was obvious that he projected his feelings of envy and jealousy into others quite successfully. The results of such mental activity were blatant in the way he imagined others to be quite envious of his beautiful 'mind-world' and would constantly attribute jealousy to all around him.

PH's problem with successfully projecting and so ridding himself of any unpleasant awareness seemed to be limited to those situations where he felt he might be about to lose his delusional cloudless world. Frequently this loss was precipitated by external events, such as being expelled from a squat, the suicide of a 'friend', or being sent to prison for some reason or other. However, such precipitating events characteristically seemed to lose their anxiety-provoking significance quite quickly. They could be mentally processed.

In the psychotherapy, the way he disposed of anxiety had to be reiterated, as it occurred, so that he could recognise what was going on and how dangerously provocative such activity could prove to be. Clinically the interesting thing was that, despite its dangerous quality, the awareness of the cause of trouble could be split off and projected apparently so easily.

I have no real idea why PH went mad in the first instance and what caused him to create and maintain his delusional cloudless world. I do think I know the contents of his delusional existence to be really satisfying and available immediately. They permitted him to recognise himself as an essential member of an important group – idolised and loved universally – and to repair his situation. The trouble is that it was inevitable that either some residual sane capacity to see reality as it was, or maybe an endogenous depressive element, would intrude and spoil it all.

By the time of his violent attacks it is my belief that one of the major intruders in this unfortunate man's life was the major tranquillising drug he had been prescribed. Such drugs intrude into the beautiful world, by sedating unconscious anxieties. This sedation of the unconscious anxieties then interfered with the formation of the psychotic dream world created to repair his mind of its feeling of utter emptiness, isolation, rejection and jealousy.

Second Patient: JP

JP assaulted a perfect stranger on the London Underground, attempting to push him off the platform. As I have mentioned, the circumstances in which I saw him allowed me to provide more in-depth treatment.

By the time I saw him he was a 60-year-old worn-out man. He had been an in-patient in a secure psychiatric hospital for fifteen years, having been admitted under a legal procedure (as a danger to the public because of what he had done) in the late 1970s. He was emphysematous and smoked incessantly. Until he got used to the possibility that he could speak to me in his sessions in an ordinary fashion, he spoke in an ordered, sycophantic and apologetic way, as if I were a superior officer, who not only demanded this but could punish him for its absence. He would agree with everything said to him – as if disagreement was dangerous.

He had waited a very long time to come to the unit (which provides a preferable environment to alternatives) and talking to me was the only means available to him to ensure his stay there and balance his unbalanced mind. He would interlace his ideas, occasionally at the onset but more frequently later, with statements from literary and dramatic sources. He was clearly well read and informed. He claimed an attachment to far left political thoughts and to Roman Catholicism. He certainly has a history of racist attitudes, and is occasionally overtly racist and superior.

JP had grown up in the North of England and is the fourth and youngest child in a coal mining family. His father, a heavy-drinking man, was described by him as having no status in the mining community. The patient himself worked underground for a year but ran away from home a year later, aged 16. He joined a circus. Later he joined a

Guards regiment, following in the footsteps of one of his older brothers. In the Guards his good record was periodically spoilt by drinking episodes, but he finished his service as a sergeant, despite a long period in detention. Various occupations and interests and wanderings followed. There are constant reports in the various notes. He was felt to be rather a good journalist and a good actor, but invariably something interfered and spoiled the situation.

The first admission took place in his late twenties – followed by a series of admissions, each terminated by apparent cures, agreement to stop drinking and promises of refusal to take drugs. He was also frequently discharged because of aggressive destructive behaviour and some violence towards staff. Throughout, the diagnoses given to this man were always almost standard ones of schizophrenia. But there had been phases where he read, worked well and published short stories and literary criticism – and some poems.

This patient has never seemed able to attach himself to anybody or anything. He was married twice. Both wives left him. He was promiscuous and there was a history of homosexual prostitution. His story about his assault at the tube station varied from the facts, as they were known to the authorities, in two essential details. Firstly, concerning the time before the attack. He originally told me that his welfare benefits were a day late in arriving and that this had worried him. Later he corrected this account. He had actually arrived at the welfare office a day late because he had been drinking heavily. He had expected that the 'nice lady' at the office would be helpful because she had always been nice to him before. In fact she was unable to help and asked him to return later, expressing doubts as to whether his money would be available. It was at the tube station later that he made the attack, having become convinced people were giving up on him. He stuck to this account throughout my treatment of him.

His experience then was that somebody who had been so helpful and kind, was giving up on him and that it was his own fault this was happening. He was angry, excited, miserable and penniless. He grabbed a man on the platform – a stranger – and pushed him towards the line, forcibly. Fortunately, although the man's legs were over the edge, he was saved from further ghastly injury.

The patient's story about these events is interesting because his account was again different from the facts and again in a very important way – given my developing thesis about these patients. He said he was convinced that his victim was trying to commit suicide. He remembered this in his sessions with me and admitted that he had great difficulty in giving up this belief. He added, in this context, that his own behaviour was designed simply to frighten the man out of such behaviour. A later version was that the man had insulted him by calling him a Jew and that this had upset him.

Actually these two versions of the story (that the man was suicidal and in need of a fright, or by thinking that our patient was a Jew, thereby insulting him), although far from each other in one sense, are not so dissimilar. In the first version he clearly projects his murderously suicidal ideas into the man who is his victim. By 'trying to frighten him' he reveals how he has split the conflict that existed in the psychotic part of his mind and has disposed of his suicidal self into his victim. In the second version, bearing in mind his racist attitudes in which Jews were considered to be degraded like blacks, the picture of himself as accused of being a Jew at the time of the attack involves the same conflict. The victim had become a split-off part of himself and was felt to be making an accusation about what he is like. Either way the victim is made to possess some very unwanted and depressing qualities compared to his idealised view of himself.

After the attack, the patient's behaviour was described as grandiose: he claimed to have won the Victoria Cross (the highest medal for bravery in the British armed forces) and seems to have justified himself by racist comments about Jews and black people.

As I see the pathology, we are here looking at the way the psychotic part of this man's mind works. In that part of his mind it is a traumatic disappointment to have any awareness that 'he feels himself to be inferior' to the person he was, before the traumatic disappointment in the welfare office. To him, to feel inferior not only faces him with his own (defective) racist ideas but also with exaggerated ideas about how intolerable this is – exaggerations derived from his split-off maniacal superiority. In this kind of psychotic functioning, projections are split off violently and suddenly and carry the need for delusional certainty. His good object, exemplified externally by the lady in the welfare office, becomes in disappointment the object of his total murderousness and these feelings towards the previously nice lady have to be got rid of very quickly. To feel suicidal or like a Jew or a black, as he conceives them, is to be subjected to a terrible catastrophic psychotic anxiety and this must be projected.

The attack served the function of a violent and totally convincing reversal. After it he felt restored to his position of superiority. He has achieved a relatively bland, hypocritical position, *vis-à-vis* the victim. He can walk away feeling all is right with his mental world. Thus, in this case as with the first one, a sense of grandeur takes place following the events. PH felt as if he had purified himself. JP felt he deserved a medal which would be recognised and responded to by the Queen. JP's grandeur was related to having overcome the threat of utter hopelessness and emptiness, but mostly it was a maniacal belief in his own omnipotence to restore a mental state, freed of any physical truth. It is not difficult to guess why he was so smug.

In fact, I believe this kind of violently active procedure is quite usual in this man's case. He has, for example, no difficulty continuing to smoke despite his crippling emphysema. He seems to feel he triumphs over this illness, not only by denying it but by treating it as a statement of inferiority in somebody else. He is free to persecute his emphysema. As with the first patient, what is again curious is the differential capacity for splitting and for projection. There is a selective separation of what can and cannot go. The disappointment at the welfare office and the subsequent events created problems of a different order. Those mental events had to be accompanied by a violent and physical projection. This seems to have been due to his mind losing the feeling of having good (albeit delusional) objects within himself. It is in this circumstance that he can't project his feeling without the physical enactment and reassurance.

To throw more light on the case, I will now describe some of the therapeutic work that was possible with the patient.

Loss and the various responses and results of it featured in the sessions with me, albeit indirectly. He would talk about what was, what had been, what could have been, what so and so said or wrote, and said and wrote no more. However, he was always protected from the actual experience of loss by a veneer of superiority, which in his everyday dealings on the unit, irritated some people. In a funny way, he resembled the previous patient. That patient lived in his delusional world with pop stars. This patient reported links with people of substance in the literary and political world which carried the sound of truth. He knew their real names and their real thoughts. He read and discussed what he read and wrote for the hospital magazine. It was quite readable material.

Gradually his childhood entered into the sessions. He could not really understand why everybody made such a fuss about the failure of his family to remain in touch with him or he with them. To him it was just a continuation of his childhood experience. He felt he was by now inured to such deprivation. For him in his own egocentric world what counted was what 'they' thought of him. I never really got to the full constitution of 'they', but he admitted that he day-dreamed all the time about him and them. He told me how he fantasised conversing and smoking and drinking with them all together. He once joked and said if he published his thoughts there would be a large market for their pornographic quality.

Clearly, with this second patient, as with the first, his dream world kept him well thought of and warmly welcomed by his private circle. Despite his being exposed by his drinking, which he seemed to use to lubricate his inner world, I felt more optimistic about this man's future than that of the first patient.

Where JP's analysis was so different from the ordinary everyday analytic situation was in the strangely restrictive world he had lived in for over four decades. I am referring in the first instance to the interferences and inroads his illness had made upon his mind – whether we refer here to what was generally believed to be the psychotic illnesses or to the long alcoholic episodes and their interference with ordinary life and ordinary life experiences. He had also been enclosed for nearly two decades in a maximum security hospital. For him the odd nature of having an analysis in a medium-secure unit was quite acceptable and easy to tolerate.

The sessions themselves had a peculiarly enclosed and enclosing character – almost a claustrophilic quality – which I felt were a reflection of his mind's penumbrated quality. Behind this he was having a long-term relationship of total privacy and primacy with his inner circle. He was the subject of interest though sometimes unfortunately only to myself. In the perverse areas of his mind this served a purpose. He could be as delinquently careless and even as mad as he liked. He always felt there was someone listening and caring about him – a situation he had otherwise never known. I was perturbed about what seemed to be the perverse quality of such behaviour. It would vary from sleepiness and inattentiveness to paroxysmal episodes of sleepiness of almost narcoleptic intensity. On the other side were periods of manic chatting and gossiping.

It was eventually possible to link these patterns to his identification (a) with his heavy drinking father and (b) his feeling of himself as like his father: a man of just the poor status and little respect which he was so busy denying via his behaviour patterns. This led me to be able to connect the perverse character of his behaviour with his period of homosexual prostitution. Then he had enjoyed not only the physical but what he called the social 'lies' of these relationships – some casual, others repetitious. As our sessions continued, gradually a more thoughtful person emerged, although even this had a quality of ambiguity and cynical jokiness. Understanding this turned out to be crucial.

In one particular session the patient had decided, on his way to the session, that he would like to, or perhaps that he would, smoke. At this point he had given up smoking during sessions. He felt that he was beginning to recognise his capacity to be provocatively aggressive because he knew that I disliked his smoking. After telling me, he became silent for a while. I was suddenly extremely doubtful about the sincerity of this presentation. I felt as if I were being invited to believe something that I would later feel foolish about having believed. I shared my doubt with him and added that he didn't know if he was being sensible or trying to please or trick me.

He replied that actually he was having difficulty in keeping me out of the 'pornographic' conversations that he had with himself. I said that he felt relieved that I had openly questioned his sincerity. I added that he was afraid of corrupting me. He did this to his own mind sometimes consciously with his fairy stories and he felt his mind to be corrupted more seriously – as had happened when he felt he had damaged the woman at the welfare office on the occasion of the assault. This time it was he himself who was not keeping his promise to himself – not to smoke – in the session.

He then spoke of his anxieties about the future. Where was he going to live and work when the sessions ended? He thought he looked like a comedian on the TV. That man could apparently distort his face so completely he could become somebody unlike himself and be the person his face was impersonating. I took this to imply he was talking about his own weird identifications and their distorting effect upon his mind and behaviour: how easily he lost his sense of 'self'.

This session was typical of the last few months of his stay in the Unit. It gave the opportunity to repeat the kind of work his illness required. His problem in sessions like this was to become aware that a joke can rebound so that he would be left feeling empty of future and purpose. In later sessions, the metaphor of the comedian was replaced by talking about the various psychiatrists he had known over the years. His experience was that they had avoided knowing about his mind and its vagaries and had instead been friendly and given him general advice. As he said to me, 'Fancy advising me!' To him such treatment had been a graphic repetition of his own previously thoughtless and somewhat condescending attitude towards himself and his mind. The attitude was at the centre of the problem of tricking, being tricked, and of trickery itself. He felt he had either tricked the doctors into stupidly believing in a potential in him, which he couldn't maintain, or that they now contained his own trickery and condescension to the extent they were now tricksters. It was for this reason that he was so relieved in the session described when I queried his sincerity. At the same time he felt life had tricked him, by giving him so many real talents but not the equipment to use them. This reflected his unhappy identification with his father – who drank and had no status but relieved this by drinking. This in turn led to his belief about why he resorted to 'pornography'. This was really only a fantasy life of constant availability of companionship, only sometimes sexual. What I took him really to be saying was that his good objects were seduced objects and seducing objects. For this reason they were bound to be both unreliable and fragile.

It was in connection with these features that we began to work through again the complications of his assault. It became understandable. Although he hated the idea, he began to see and feel the need for seriousness. He ended treatment with an awareness of his aggressive behaviour and potential and its role in how the assault had come about. He asked, 'Was I born insane, or did something make me insane?' I suppose the answer is yes, you had a predilection – though I never knew all about his earliest years – and, yes, to the second part too. He also knew that there were times when the only thing that interested him was drinking. Maybe it would have been more profitable if we had met thirty years earlier. Certainly in the course of our meetings he had become actually interested in himself in the sessions – not in his usual narcissistic fashion but introspectively and seriously in the actual person.

Third Patient: ME

ME is 30 years old and was born in the West Indies. He also assaulted someone on a tube station: this time it was a tourist, who was actually pushed on to the line.

ME came to the hospital from prison in a floridly psychotic state. It was not long after the assault and he was dirty and dishevelled, tense and highly aroused. He was irritable and unwilling to discuss his previous psychiatric history. There were also frequent 'clang' associations, e.g. 'The mental hospital with the dental mechanic'. He appeared to be distressed by paranoid ideation as when he said 'Why don't you kill me and grind my bones?'

At the time of the assault, and for a while after, he had totally denied its occurrence. However, by the time I saw him, he was able to acknowledge that something had happened and to tell me that he felt entitled to say that he had not pushed his victim: it was as if something had jumped out of him and hit the man. Gradually the details of his account came to coalesce with the truth and he could remember assaulting the man on the platform. From the point of view of the theme developed with the other two patients, his first description is, of course, most interesting.

During his sessions with me, ME was predominantly concerned with ideas on two themes: the loss of his job, for which he had trained so hard and in which he had done so well, and the way he felt mocked by the man who sacked him and how depressed he became as a result. However, this man did have a history of previous delinquent aggressive behaviour. On one occasion he had assaulted a policeman and on another an unknown man.

ME's anger featured considerably in his talks with me. His fury at the world could, he felt, manifest itself at the slightest sign of what he called being 'frustrated'. Gradually I learned that these frustrations referred to some thought or other which he did not recognise and to three traumatic occasions: (a) his being hooked out of the West Indies to live in the UK; (b) the loss of his job; and (c) his original loss of his mother.

After initially welcoming and liking the idea, ME resented seeing me and talking to me about himself. He wanted to have nothing to do with the things to which I referred. He wished to be free of them. When listening to him, I found I could clearly differentiate the paranoid psychotic phases in his life and his account from the events leading up to the situation on the tube station. His experience was that he had been something and then he was nothing. His innocent victim was obviously a tourist and looked happy. Undoubtedly this was what ME felt to be so provocative. The tourist was without a care and lived in a carefree careless world. The pattern of events described with the other two patients, following the loss of good objects, followed.

For this patient, his good object was his work, about which he held what seemed to be a justifiable sense of pride. This, he felt, had been totally ignored when he had lost his position when the firm retrenched and made a group of the staff redundant. He felt particularly badly treated at receiving summary dismissal. Until then there had been no complaints about his performance and he now felt he was suddenly being told he was not good enough to be kept on. Such cruel treatment, he reasoned, could only be explained, possibly correctly, because he was black.

In his sessions, the patient protected himself valiantly from any experience of being easily dischargeable and redundant. He was infuriatingly condescending and superior and he regularly gave me notice that he would not attend, or would terminate his sessions.

His history and development seemed to guarantee such a defence system. Unfortunately, like that of the offspring of so many Caribbean emigrants, what had happened to him was specific. He was abandoned by his mother in his fifteenth month. Then, until the age 15, he lived with his grandmother before emigrating to the UK to rejoin his family, arriving in a bitterly cold winter and feeling he had lost his granny totally against his will.

At school he had done reasonably well and he had gone through an apprenticeship and worked well after qualification at his trade. He described to me his problems at his first English school. He had to sit on his hands, because he had no means of knowing what to do with them. In the West Indies he just knew he had promising hands, good hands.

There had been one admission to a mental hospital prior to the index offence. Then he was described as over-active with poor personal hygiene and aggressive and difficult to manage although previously he had been described as a shy introverted man – there was a suggestion of heavy cannabis abuse.

Losing his job, after such care and nurture, confirmed for ME how dangerously easy it was to have a devastating mental loss and, like JP, he was an aggressive man, fertile soil for the developments I've described.

Discussion

The view I take about these three patients, which I believe equally true about any of the others in the series, is that their diagnoses were incorrect. They are not schizophrenics but the victims of mixed conditions in which total intolerance for any depressive experience leads to a need to act out physically. Such patients can be differentiated from those with other mixed states by virtue of their life histories, in which loss has been totally and psychotically denied. If they are exposed endogenously and possibly externally to such losses, such people and the public are dangerously and unnecessarily exposed. I have commented on the dangers that major tranquillising drugs can introduce into this situation.

These three men have another characteristic: they are almost but not quite importunate, they are 'dying' to talk to somebody. I found them approachable and responsive to talk. They would, in effect, tell me what was going on inside them quite easily, although they are not really aware of the significance of what they are saying. They are, therefore, lost souls waiting for somebody to care for them: they seldom find care except in the psychotic parts of their minds. This state of being lost fluctuates and can be replaced by rebellious resistance and absenting.

The perception of self is the inner self's view of its own reputation. In these patients, any mood changes, irritability and a sense of total dissatisfaction with self, and its converse manic happiness, and dramatic story-telling, have to be noted as dangerous prognostic signs, which means the need for repetitive mental state examinations during the course of therapy, but particularly during ongoing care. Their minds and the emotional contents of them are the barometers of change and have to be noted.

In these patients, there is an angry experience that responds to the loss of their previous mental state, which each man in his own way considered as happiness. In response to loss, they all found what they believed to be, and later denied, a non-depressed 'non-caring' person who became a 'suitable victim'. Prior to their assault, each of them felt that an unprovoked attack had taken place within himself, and following their responses to such an inner assault, even felt themselves to be honourably restored. It was only much later that each was invited to know that he had been mad and had attacked somebody other than himself.

This short summary also summarises the aims of treatment: to provide them with an awareness of their actual and potential aggressiveness; of their hopelessness and despair at the delusional loss of their 'good' inner world; and of their anger towards, and the precarious balance of their relationship towards, the external representatives of the psychotic inner world. All of this implies, after an exciting honeymoon when the patient may be available in the early days of treatment, that resentment, suspicion and distrust will come to colour their attitude towards prolonged treatment and make future treatment in the community precarious at best, and considerably anxiety-provoking at worst.

At a theoretical and intrapsychic level the questions these cases raise are fundamental: why is there either a discriminatory or selective capacity for psychological projection, why is there an incapacity for ridding the mind of a particular form of depression? Concrete thinking and the use of violent projective mechanisms are very commonly found in schizophrenics and other severely disturbed individuals, in what ways are there specific differences in this group?

I think the first two features which start to differentiate these patients can be seen on reviewing their history. Firstly, there is no evidence of sublimation of aggressive instincts to the extent of a disturbance which may have interfered with development of the capacity for full symbolisation. Secondly, the lives of these men have been punctuated by a profound series of losses, real or imagined.

How do such patients manage projection? A symbol representing the original internal idea is produced but it is felt to be installed elsewhere than in their own minds. In JP's case he created a symbol of being free from even unconscious awareness of his murderousness to his object (the nice lady at the Welfare). This 'symbol' is represented by the appearance of suicidal ideas in the mind of the victim. Put in another way, one may view the delusion as a symbol of a successful projection.

I am suggesting that in all these patients there is a defective symbolisation of 'loss'. Because of the unsublimated state of their aggressive instincts and the inhibition of the activity that initiates symbol formation, projection or projective identification cannot take place in the usual way. I have a suspicion that the absence of an original object into which they could project feelings exaggerates this inhibition and increases the need for violent physical muscularity, to replace the failed projection. Were such symbolisation possible, projections would take place and therefore no violence would occur.

If there is concretisation in these patients, it seems to me to be specifically to keep the good objects *in* concretely, and this hardly facilitates splitting of the mind and later projection. Segal's work on symbolism (Segal, 1958, postscript 1981) and on depression in the schizophrenic (Segal, 1956) are central to my thinking about these patients. In the latter paper she states 'The thesis of this paper is that, in the course of development, schizophrenics reach the depressive position, and finding it intolerable, deal with it by projecting ... a large part of their ego into an object, that is by projective identification'. She continues, 'this is a phase of development in which the infant's ego is integrated enough ... for the infant to experience a whole object relation involving ambivalence, dread of loss, guilt and the urge to regain and restore the object.' She adds that by projective identification she means 'that process in which a part of the ego is split off and projected into an object with a consequent loss of that part of the ego, as well as an alteration in the perception of the object'.

My patients situation differed from that described by Segal. Her patient had the capacity to project a large part of the ego and its contents. this my patient could not and did not do. Like Segal's patient my patients did project their sanity, to protect their (delusional) good

72

objects. This raises a central question: is the depressive position, with the contents described by Segal, anything akin to the depressive qualities experienced by my patients? Her patient and my patients both dreaded loss, but in the situation I describe, the threat of loss was not located in the depressive position – it was experienced in a profoundly paranoid way. In the depressive position the capacity for projection is linked to the urge to regain and restore the object. Ambivalence, a central feature of the depressive position, does not interfere with the capacity to project. In a chronically schizophrenic mind the depressive position is not, clinically, a depressive illness. the disagreement between us then may be only of terminology. Depression and the depressive position are not the same. the three patients I describe frequently projected elements of the depressive position into me.

In 'Notes on symbol formation' (Segal, 1957), Segal states 'Symbol formation is an activity of the ego attempting to deal with anxieties stirred by its relation to the object and is generated by the fear of bad objects and the fear of the loss or inaccessibility of good objects. Disturbance in the ego's relation to objects are reflected in disturbances of symbol formation ... disturbances in the differentiation between ego and object lead to disturbances in differentiation between the symbol and the object symbolised and therefore to concrete thinking characteristic of psychoses'. My patients were faced with the horrifying threat of a double loss: a) the loss of their good objects and b) the loss of their capacity to get rid of this threat. The absence of the capacity to produce, psychologically, an adequate symbolic expression of this situation provides the key to the enactment that took place. The ensuing mania, in all cases, provided, as I understand it, the reassurance that now everything is as it (madly) should be.

Segal's patient A was a schizophrenic in a mental hospital. When asked, by his doctor why he had stopped playing his violin, he replied 'Why? Do you expect me to masturbate in public?' For him, she states, the violin had become so completely equated with his genitals, that to touch it in public became impossible. Put in the same position and asked 'Why didn't you project your fear of loss into the man and walk away?', the answer of my patients would have to be: 'I can't project the experience of loss. If I did I would empty my mind and myself completely.' If they were asked 'Who was the person you attacked?', the answer would have to be: 'He was what I was, before I became what I am'. And to the question 'What did he then become?': 'He became what I was'. 'And you, what did you become?' 'I became what I was before'.

In Segal's terms, the act of violence itself, therefore, is a truly symbolic equation. Copyright © Institute of Psycho-Analysis.

Acknowledgement

A earlier version of this paper was published in 1995.

Notes

1. The Denis Hill Unit is a 15-bedded unit in the grounds of the Royal Bethlem Hospital which is part of the joint Bethlem/Maudsley Hospitals. It is a medium secure unit in the care of the forensic unit of the combined hospitals. Medium-Secure Units were created to give care and security in a clinical situation halfway between locked wards and maximum security hospitals. In the case of our patients, all had become involved because of mental illness, needing the care and security of the Unit as their environment. The average length of stay is 18 months. Maximum Security Units are self-explanatory and exist for long-stay care of psychotic patients who have committed violent crimes and therefore, because of their dangerousness, long-standing care is required.

2. Courts may decide, following psychiatric advice, to remove the accused from the penal system to specific medical care, which is arranged by a variety of orders appropriate to the offence and to the patient's mental state.

3. Accommodation that has fallen vacant which groups of otherwise homeless people take over until removed by the authorities.

References

Segal, H. (1956) 'Depression in the schizophrenic', *International Journal of Psycho-Analysis*, 37: 339-43.

—— (1957) 'Notes on symbol formation', *International Journal of Psycho-analysis*, 38: 391-7.

—— (1980) Postscript to 'Notes on Symbol Formation' in (1981) *The Work of Hanna Segal*. New York: Jason Aronson.

3

Putting the Boot In

Violent Defences Against Depressive Anxiety

Robin Anderson

Introduction

In this chapter I wish to explore the use of a particular kind of violence that is brought into operation in certain patients when they experience a psychic situation which brings to awareness feelings of depressive guilt and anxiety. My central point is that unless the analyst becomes aware of the extent of this violence, and the defensive function it serves, the analysis reaches a state of stasis or impasse. To analyse this situation effectively, it is necessary for the analyst to be aware of what may appear to be quite subtle improvements in the quality of the patient's contact with his objects; and, also, to understand the enormous difficulties the patient encounters in maintaining this improved state.

I term this type of violence 'putting the boot in', as this captures the quality of the primitive, almost mindless, violence which serves, I believe, to annihilate an object felt to be damaged and vulnerable. This expression refers to a situation in a fight where one party falls to the ground, is clearly beaten, and may even appeal for mercy. 'Putting the boot in' has a resonance for finishing off the helpless opponent. I use this term also as it fits so well with the fantasies of the patient whom I will describe.

Hanna Segal has made the distinction between depressive pain and guilt as a persecution, as opposed to the quality of depressive pain which can be experienced as sadness, longing and regret. The defence against depressive anxiety which is expressed as violence against an object is also an outcome of a disturbance in the capacity to perceive an object as separate from the self. In a paper called 'What is the object, the role of perception', Segal (1990) emphasises the change that takes place in the capacity to perceive an object in the move between the paranoid schizoid and the depressive positions. In the paranoid schizoid position, projective identification dominates the picture and the distinction between the self and the object is either indistinct or is based not on the reality of separation but on the degree to which the self wishes to be rid of some unwanted part of itself.

In 'Acting on Fantasy and Acting on Desire' (1992), Segal describes violent defences against perception and vulnerability in the self which take the form of attacks on an object felt to contain unwanted and unbearable parts of the self. She gives an example of a forensic case where a child had been murdered. The child was murdered at the point when he became frightened and started crying. The murderer did not know why he did this. As a small child, he had been abused and had been terrified and lonely. At the age of 3, he had tried to kill himself. In his analysis

> ... it quickly became apparent that the little boy was perceived by the man as though he was himself as a small child, and when he became frightened, lonely, and started to cry, it was intolerable to the man, as was the memory of himself in the same state of mind as a little boy. His suicidal impulse at the age of 3 became the compulsive murder of the little boy, seen as a child in himself who had to be killed.

I believe a process very similar to this is at work in the type of patient I will describe (though taking place intrapsychically) where what is attacked is not simply a hostile object, but a vulnerable and suffering part of the self which it is felt imperative to silence.

Clinical Example

I would like to describe one such patient in his very early and tentative moves towards being able to experience and own depressive anxiety.

The patient, a man in his mid-30s, had been in analysis with me for some years before the period I wish to describe. His original complaints were of long-standing depression, unhappiness, inability to progress in his life, and difficulties in relationships with others, particularly with women. The patient was brought up in another country, but moved to England with his family when he was very young. Although there was no material impoverishment, there was considerable evidence of a very emotionally impoverished childhood, although there was no history, as far as I could discern, of any major childhood trauma.

This was, however, something I could never feel certain about. When he was 8 or 9, his father suffered a mild stroke and, following this, remained somewhat depressed and fearful that it might recur. The patient, however, had shown signs of disturbance before this. He was the eldest of four children, three boys and a younger girl; it was difficult to get a sense of his life as a child although he conveyed a family atmosphere that was harsh, depriving and cold. There was intense competition between him and his brothers for their powerful mother's affection. However, later in the analysis, the picture seemed less extreme, and it was difficult to be certain as to the true nature of the situation.

He hated reaching puberty and was subsequently very sexually inhibited. When he first presented in analysis he had never had any sexual experience other than masturbation. His masturbation was frequently accompanied by putting on boots and looking at himself in a mirror. Boots were an important preoccupation for him. He admired them and acquired many different varieties: army boots, police boots, riding boots, cowboy boots, etc. There were often links between the boots and violent sadistic and very powerful men like Hitler and the Nazis, Stalin, Saddam Hussein; and sometimes less obviously tyrannical figures like policemen, soldiers, horse-riders, or motorcyclists.

Though he maintained that his masturbatory activity made him feel manly, this never felt entirely convincing. He never could be really excited or satisfied by it, but this perverse activity united him, in fantasy, with an object which gave him a feeling of having a protective covering, like a kind of rubber or leather skin. This covering dulled his anxiety but gave him little satisfaction, and this became clear, as I will later show, in the way this activity was manifested in the transference. He was as much imprisoned in this situation as rescued by it. Although his fantasy world was full of violence and cruelty, he had never in fact acted this out externally, and had never been physically violent. However, his feelings towards those he felt had slighted him (his parents, his colleagues at work, and his analyst) were extreme, unforgiving and full of hatred.

During the early years of his analysis, he had made some progress, but this was most apparent in his professional life. Having been almost unable to function at work because of his shyness and awkwardness, resulting in the loss of several jobs, he had become an increasingly successful scientist, and was professionally well regarded. He was more successful socially, less isolated, and had a few friends. Since the break with a girlfriend two years previously he had not embarked on any other close relationship. In fact the relationship to his previous girlfriend was the only one that he had ever had.

In working with him I became increasingly aware of a particular atmosphere that had a powerful effect on me, and on him too. I will illustrate this by bringing some fairly typical material.

He arrived a few minutes late for a Monday session, looking rather grey and unsmiling. He began:

> The weekend was awful. What could anyone expect, as I have no girlfriend? Without a girlfriend there isn't any point to anything. I did almost nothing – all the things I had intended to do, like studying, producing food for the party, cleaning my flat – none of them. I haven't seen anyone except my parents ... how devastating to be in my 30s and only have my parents to go and see ... They have so much to answer for – to have been treated so terribly as a child and with such a cold mother. Then my father spoke about homosexuals at his hairdresser and I knew by the way he spoke that he just can't cope with homosexuality ... Anyway, what's the point in coming here? You can't deal with my problems. I think you're not up to it. In fact, if it wasn't for the fact that I know you give lectures I would be absolutely convinced that you aren't capable of working with me. I don't know whether I'm too much for you, or my case is just too difficult.

And so it went on, an all-too-familiar unfolding of a kind of commentary which I tried to work with, and think about. It was difficult to have any conviction that these accounts arose from a desire for this situation to be any different. Indeed, he became convinced that he did not believe this was a possibility. Although he clearly felt hopeless, there did not seem to be a real desire for understanding; only a wish to nurse this aggrieved state. As this awareness dawned in me it was hard not to have a sense of indignation. In trying to think about interpreting this situation it felt very hard to avoid a countertransference enactment in which my interpretation would simply be a thinly-disguised expression of indignation which would be likely to lead to an impasse, with an aggrieved patient and analyst complaining to each other.

His way of relating conveyed a feeling that any goodness was absent, indeed had never been present. It created a sense of lifelessness in the room which was most disturbing. It was possible to observe that this material was not motivated by a wish to convey the truth of his situation but more by a desire to induce feelings, both in the object and in himself, of despair and paralysis. This activity was carried out with such conviction and forcefulness that they became reality for him, and very often for me too. I was at times aware of a kind of relish which this hold over reality gave him, and this provided some evidence of the underlying sadism and violence.

78

By this activity he locked himself into his object, creating an insepa-rable couple united in a kind of loveless sadistic marriage. This claustrophobic situation was one which meant that interpretation could not be made with any sense of conviction, and from the patient's point of view was probably felt to be the analyst's attempt to escape from an unbearable situation.

I think the maintenance of this position was closely linked to the patient's perverse masturbatory activity which I described earlier, in which he and his object were fused in a grim rubberised togetherness, based on cruelty and violence. In this sadomasochistic intercourse the distinction between self and object was obliterated in the patient's mind. In this way he was psychically married to an object which he kept in a subjugated and depressed state.

As I tried to explore the situation further, I became aware of a number of factors that affected it. Any forward movement increased the intensity of his need violently to constrict his object, preventing any awareness of the object's independence of him. I think this was a reaction to a separation between himself and the analyst when he was faced with his analyst's independence from him, provoking a violent reaction which served to re-establish the old equilibrium once more. When it was possible to see what was happening, and to interpret it without the enactment of retaliation, he was enormously relieved, and at these points it was possible to detect an abrupt change in the atmosphere of the session that was very striking.

This powerful tyranny over the object seemed to obliterate the possibility of any enquiry into the state of the object, or of any interest in it, or even knowledge of it, and so served as a powerful defence against depressive anxiety. But this manoeuvre was felt additionally to damage the object, with resultant guilt, producing even greater perse-cution. Any real facing of the state of the object remained an almost insuperable task.

This more overtly violent relation to a damaged object, 'putting the boot in', was illustrated in some later material.

It was the first day back after a public holiday, and I had forgotten to unlock the entry door to my rooms. As a result, the door failed to open when I pressed the lock release, so that the patient was denied his usual 'automatic entry', and had to wait until I unlocked the door. I knew that this was likely to cause a reaction – perhaps for several weeks. I became somewhat preoccupied with this, and in a slightly flustered way I accidentally set off my watch alarm at the end of the session. He seemed somewhat less upset than I had expected, and the next day he brought a dream in which

> a bumble-bee had got into his home. He had mixed feelings about this bee: on the one hand he hated it and feared it would sting him and should be killed; on the other, that it was trapped and wanted only to be able to follow its natural instincts to get out and pollinate flowers, collect nectar, and breed.
>
> He began to kill it by hitting it repeatedly, but after five or six blows he was surprised to notice that it was more resilient than he had expected (he described it as 'tougher' and therefore less squashable than he had thought) and he wished he had not started to kill it. But now he had started, he felt he had to continue; because otherwise it would be left injured and he could not bear to let that happen.

The dream seemed to demonstrate how he could not stop his violent, damaging activity, not only because of his sadistic gratification, but just as importantly because he would have to stop and face what he had done; and so he went on with the killing. It may be that this process was initiated by some sense of an already-damaged object as manifest in this material by my forgetful and bumbling behaviour on that day. However, I think the capacity to bring a dream was in itself an indication of some development of a more resilient (less squashable) and therefore less persecutory internal object. He had (to his surprise) survived better over that Bank Holiday weekend, and now he was confronted by his violent defence against depressive anxiety – a continuous 'putting the boot in', the awareness of which pained him and necessitated an intensification of the defence.

Some further understanding of his tendency to exaggerate and over-emphasise any slights and setbacks in his life became possible some time after this.

He arrived at a subsequent session and reported a 'disaster'. A junior technician where he worked, a woman, played squash with him. On the way to the court she had said 'I hope you don't hit me'. He was very angry that anyone should suggest such a thing, and was then 'outraged' and 'devastated' when she hit him in the mouth with her racquet and broke his front tooth. This clearly disturbing event now became the nucleus of a grievance which was becoming more and more exaggerated. He was furious with her and said he 'realised' that this was an 'envious attack' by her, and he thought of suing her. He had a conviction that his looks were now permanently spoiled and so the small chance he had to be married had now been taken away for ever. He brought a dream in which

> he was enlarging a photograph. In association he mentioned an art exhibition he had recently visited. The artist had produced a photo, vastly enlarged (thirty feet long) of a crater. He had then altered the crater, enlarging it further with dynamite, and produced a second vast photograph.

This sense of a vast enlargement of the damage to his tooth illustrated rather clearly his relationship to damage and defect in himself (and in his objects). He involved himself in a process of vast enlargement and exaggeration, and then displayed them for all the world (especially his analyst) to see. He made a work of art out of the defects, for which he felt the objects were to blame, and this became the main interest in his life, taking precedence over, and helping him ignore, the awful state of his own inner world and his part in its creation. (In fact, he reported the next day that his dentist had made a 'beautiful repair' of his tooth.) By the same token the enlargement meant that he had far more to face because everything he did, as well as what was done to him, became so exaggerated. I felt too that this process was related to his masturbatory activity, as though the boots made him enormous and eradicated all feelings of smallness and helplessness.

He was quite shaken, but was able to listen when I interpreted this to him. I found that something had shifted in my own position and that I was less preoccupied with escaping from being trapped, and more trying to convey to him what I felt to be true and helpful to him – a shift from a paranoid schizoid to a depressive countertransference position, which felt strengthening to me.

I think it was clear from this material that a quite different way of relating to the object had become possible. He had been able to allow me to emerge from a position in which I was trapped and constricted by him, to a position in which I felt able to move and talk to him. He then became able to listen to the disturbing interpretations, and this resulted in there being a gap between us.

How could this be possible for him? I think that when he heard the analyst making sense to him of his experience he did feel that there was a 'beautiful repair', not only of himself but of his object as well, and this was enormously reassuring to him when he lived in a world populated by damaged blaming and persecuting objects. For this reason I believe he could tolerate the disturbing aspects of the contact – the narcissistic wound.

81

I think that in the world of 'locked-in', 'rubberised' relationships, where there was no real object, he was deprived even of the awareness of an understanding object, so that when he could discern that he was being understood this did also satisfy a longing in him for a different kind of relationship that he had lost contact with: when the analyst had found a way of freeing himself from this entanglement then he could experience an object that could be responsive to him and thoughtful about him and could allow him to feel helped. This new experience was deeply gratifying to him.

It became more apparent, therefore, that his difficulties were principally derived from his fear of a perception of damaged objects – a situation that is similar but in fact quite distinct from the situation where violence is stimulated by envy.

Returning to the clinical material, I now want to give some detailed material from a session in the period leading up to the summer holiday. The improvement in his condition had been sustained, and was accompanied by the emergence of a quite distinct type of depression which was less persecuting, and involved a greater capacity to experience loss with accompanying sadness. Although there was frequently the emergence of an aggressive quality in the sessions, this was much more open and accompanied by the sense of freedom and movement in the analysis.

He had previously tended to arrive a few minutes late for his sessions, but he was now occasionally coming early, and was thus confronted with having to wait. This capacity to wait, I thought, was linked to his capacity to tolerate my separateness. As he was the first patient of the day, and I work at home, this meant a confrontation with me upstairs with my family. I felt this capacity was a concrete expression of his tolerance of my thinking, being upstairs with the family in my mind.

I wish to give a detailed report of a Thursday session. However, I will first briefly outline some of the events which had occurred in the session on the previous day.

He had arrived early, and continued for much of the session complaining that I could not work with him because I obviously did not like him since I had greeted him in such an unfriendly way. He had the conviction that I was not pleased to see him despite the fact that he had made the effort to come early. Eventually I discovered that he had been disturbed by the slight delay in my pressing the lock-release button. (This delay would not have occurred if he had arrived late, as I would normally have been in the consulting-room and near to the button; however, his arriving early meant I was upstairs in my house and further from a lock-release button.) At the end of that session he had been able to make the unusual acknowledgement that he knew that just because he had felt those things about me did not mean that they were true. In this way, he was showing how he had developed a capacity to have a perspective on himself: to have a view and also to hold on to the idea of a different view, thus to identify with the analyst's capacity to see things differently from the way he was seeing them himself.

The following day, he arrived four minutes late again, and wondered if it had to do with the 'tiny delay' yesterday (note the lack of exaggeration). He had forgotten his pager as well, but he said this was not too serious and would certainly not lead to a patient's investigation being delayed, though it might lead any junior doctor trying to reach him to wonder what on earth had happened. I pointed out that he had managed to hold onto the fact that it had been a *small delay* yesterday, but he had nonetheless wanted to make the junior doctor suffer by wondering what had happened, just as he had been left wondering what had happened to me yesterday.

He then spoke of his anger with his professor over his holiday plans. He had been put on a duty rota when he was supposed to be at a conference, and his professor should have remembered that. He did realise that the professor was very busy, but he had told him of his plans. I connected this with an attempt to be more flexible with me over my holiday plans, which did not coincide with his own arrangements. (He had previously made some holiday arrangements which meant he would have to re-start his analysis one week late and had threatened to leave his analysis unless I altered my holiday dates.) Now he was saying that he realised he had never discussed his own plans with me; so it was not really fair of him to go on at me about it.

He had had a dream in which

he was in a room like mine, consulting a woman doctor about a virus infection he had contracted. She was not taking his infection seriously enough. He had a chicken-pox-like rash, and he noticed he had some vesicles in his eyes. He remembered in the dream that he had already had chicken-pox. Could it have been shingles? If so, to get it so young could mean that he must have a disturbance in his immune system. Did this mean he had AIDS or leukaemia? Should he therefore take a modest anti-viral agent or a more powerful and dangerous one? He was not sure.

Then he reported a second dream, in which

a man drove up in a yellow Mini to consult him about a rabies risk. This man was either going on his holiday to a risky area, or had just returned from one, but he needed this to be properly looked at and resolved.

An association to the yellow Mini was his neighbour, an old man, who had recently died. He was actually not poor, but drove a Mini because he was a very unpretentious man – not the type to drive around in a Rolls Royce, even if he had the money, because he had different values. He would rather have a photograph of his grandchildren, or books on world wild-life. (In a session not long before this, he had also spoken of the neighbour as a man who could live on his own, because, although he had lost his wife, he had loved her and the memory of this could sustain him, even though he was now without her.) At this point the patient paused, and looked at his watch – there were ten more minutes – and said 'I have another association, rather a lengthy one'. He then launched into a long and involved account of a rabies call that he had had recently. He reached a point in the story where the consultant had rightly decided that there had been some urgency and had insisted that the vaccine must be sent Express.

I broke in and suggested that there was an infection that needed urgent treatment, and that it could not wait till the next day. I suggested that the infection that could flare up was due to my small delay the day before, which had affected his way of looking at me in his mind's eye. The vesicles meant that he was aware that something had happened in that 'look', that he had hated me when he 'saw' me with my family upstairs. He did not know how seriously he had damaged me, but he struggled to restore me – to remember me as a good man who holds onto a picture of the child/himself; but there were painful things about this 'good' man: he had died, and when he was alive he had been sad because he missed his wife and was old and infirm. So it was hard to hold onto this good but painful picture, and he was tempted to go off into his own expertise and silence me in the last minutes of the session, instead of allowing a modest treatment that might help him to recover his health. He remained silent but thoughtful for the last few minutes of the session.

Comment on the Material

I think that the fluctuations in that session show something of the struggle this patient engaged in just on the threshold of the depressive position.

He had arrived at the session in a better state, aware that my 'crime', and perhaps his own, was not too serious; it had not become exaggerated in his mind and the delay had remained a 'tiny one'. I think his association about the forgotten pager being 'not too serious' was also some measure of this. He could allow himself (the hospital doctor) to wonder what on earth had happened to me, without succumbing to overwhelming guilt and persecution. Indeed, he could allow himself to have an object about which he was curious.

I think at this point I did not understand him so well, and the interpretation that he had wished to make the hospital doctor suffer was probably not only incorrect but was also aggressive. Maybe I put the boot into him. He followed my interpretation with a criticism of the professor for 'not remembering', though he held on to a sense of proportion about this – 'the professor is very busy'. Through the dream he attempted to restore a damaged good object and to stay in relation to it, but it was too painful for him, and when he launched off with the 'long association' I think he was rapidly losing contact with me as a functioning partner. He left it to me to re-establish contact, namely not to sink back in a dead and despairing way, and in this way to rescue the situation. My wish to interpret the dream I think was evidence of my being able to hold on to the wish to restore the damage done to his object and his response shows that he was able to tolerate this and to have contact restored.

The emergence of a sense of loss, of mourning even, made further appearances. The following week, at the end of a session, he looked up at some flowers in the consulting-room and said they reminded him of the flowers that his girlfriend had given him when they had finally parted – he had tried to preserve them, to keep them alive as long as possible, but eventually, when they had died, he felt he had completely lost her.

Discussion

I think that at this moment, through his experience of sadness at the death of the flowers, he was in touch with an experience of knowing that he had not been able to keep a good object alive, and that he had been helpless to prevent this situation. The capacity to face the death of the object is so much at he heart of the depressive position. With his relentless dulling of his sensitivity, he wards off the unbearable experience. Then he and I feel as dead as the flowers that he could not keep alive; but when he becomes able to face the loss, and experience something of the despair, there is a radical alteration in the atmosphere.

Both he and I feel moved, sad, yet alive. This captures the paradox of the depressive position, so well described by Melanie Klein:

> Thus while grief is experienced to the full and despair is at its height the love for the object wells up and the mourner feels more strongly that life inside and outside will go on after all and that the lost object can be preserved within. At this stage in mourning suffering can become productive (Klein, 1940, p. 360).

It is only by facing the complete loss of the object, the inability ever to repair it, that it becomes possible for the self to feel alive rather than existing in an inert and dead state, that is in projective identification with the dead object. The persistence of this identification prevents the possibility of any separation from the object.

As I have suggested, the extreme difficulty for this patient was that any degree of separation immediately confronted him with unbearable guilt as to the state of the object, and it was only when he could have the experience of a stronger and more resilient object that he could begin to tolerate separation and the feeling of persecution could begin to diminish. In my patient the guilt arose not only from his attacks upon the object but also through the attacks on his own vulnerable self. Rosenfeld (1971) described how the destructive self, identified with an omnipotent object, captures and holds hostage, through a mixture of bullying and seduction, the libidinal or needy self, and this prevents the libidinal self from forming a dependent, creative, although sometimes painful, relationship to a good object. The material presented shows how it is not only the object that is attacked but also the capacity to see what has happened. The dream of the viral infection shows how it is the eyes that are attacked, and I think that is ultimately where the boot is put in. It is this which feels so violent. When I represent a perceiving, seeing object for him it is his own/my soft eyes which he must destroy, and he sets about this with such ferocity that at times I cannot see, or even remember what it was like to see. It is from this situation that the unbearable guilt arises, and from which he retreats into his perversion to evade or avoid any danger of seeing and suffering.

When he feels that his object's sight can recover from and resist such attacks, his sense of guilt lessens and he can then for limited periods allow himself and his object to see more clearly. His own capacity to look, however, still remains limited, as the unbearable guilt is so easily aroused.

I believe his use of his eyes and his sense of their being damaged is similar to the situation Bion refers to in his writings about psychotic processes, but occurring nearer to depressive function. With this dream, the patient brings for analysis his sense that his eyes are used to attack his objects – the old man who had died, who had lost his wife – evidence of his attack on my greater liveliness, or my 'family upstairs'. Bion has pointed out that when the psychotic patient withdraws a projection it must be withdrawn by the same organ through which the projection passed. In the situation with this patient I think it is that when the patient stops putting the boot into the analyst's eyes he is then confronted by a concrete expression of the pain of seeing his object, i.e. it is now his own damaged eyes, a kind of melancholic identification with the damaged object. In this case, my patient began to have some confidence that he has a livening and stronger object, and was thus able to begin to bear the pain of what he had done.

Conclusion

Through this account of the evolution taking place in a patient's analysis, I have tried to show how by giving importance to very small changes it was possible to begin to see how the patient's extreme and apparently mindless destruction, was serving an important defensive and therefore protective purpose. Hanna Segal has shown how depressive phenomena exist in patients who might otherwise be felt to be firmly locked in paranoid schizoid functions. At this stage, guilt is experienced as a persecutory experience from which some patients try desperately to escape. I believe that the link with a damaged object became in my patient a chain which threatened to shackle him for ever to a dead or dying object, and from which he retreated into his deadening perversion.

When it became possible for me to see some purpose in this, and indeed to sympathise with the patient's predicament, then it was possible to recover some analytic functions rather than simply to live out the patient's endless purgatory. Such a change began to bring some hope to the patient, and it was possible to begin to reverse the endless cycle of annihilation of the object (putting the boot in). Such patients can then be given hope that using, rather than destroying, their own and their objects' capacities to see and feel will offer them a surer relief from anxiety and persecution than is offered by their ultimately cold and lonely defences.

Acknowledgement

This is a new version of a previously published paper.

References

Klein, M. (1940) 'Mourning and its relation to manic-depressive states', *International Journal of Psycho-Analysis*, 21.

Riviere, J. (1936) 'A Contribution to the Analysis of the Negative Therapeutic Reaction', *International Journal of Psycho-Analysis*, 17: 304-20.

Rosenfeld, H.A. (1971) 'A clinical approach to the psychoanalytic theory of the life and death instincts: an investigation into the aggressive aspects of narcissism', *International Journal of Psycho-Analysis*, 52: 169-78.

Steiner, J. (1993) 'Two Types of Pathological Organisation in Oedipus the King and Oedipus at Colonus', in *Psychic Retreats*. London: Routledge.

Segal, H. (1990) 'What is an object? The role of perception', *Bulletin European Psychoanalytic Federation*, 35: 49-57.

—— (1992) 'Acting on Phantasy and Acting on Desire' in Hopkins, J. and Savile, A., eds, *Psychoanalysis, Mind and Art*. Oxford: Blackwell.

4

Meaning and Meaningfulness

Touching the Untouchable

Eric Brenman

In this paper I shall describe a patient with whom there was enormous difficulty in establishing shared understanding which carried convincing meaning to both analysand and analyst. Vast areas of his life appeared to be untouchable. Whilst he yearned for a relationship, he marshalled his forces to prevent being known. I hope to show a change in which this 'no go' area was reached and modified, so that he could be 'touched'. It was only after he had been in analysis for over two years that he discovered that he had suffered from severe early infantile eczema. In my view, over and above the eczema itself, the way this had been dealt with both externally and internally, appeared to have had a profound influence on the patient's capacity to evaluate what was meaningful.

I had seen this forty-five-year-old man for consultation some three months before the analysis began. He then emphasised that he suffered greatly from a depression, characterised by feelings of futility and meaninglessness in which there was no will to live. He had in the past found refuge in his work which had always remained worthwhile, and in which he had felt appreciated and rewarded by his employers. Now, most dreaded of all, the feeling of meaninglessness was invading his work; he felt that he was plunging into total hopelessness. This fear brought him to analysis. At the time I had told him that I was not certain that I would have a vacancy for him and offered to explore the possibility of an analysis for him elsewhere. He politely pressed me to make room for him.

In this initial interview I learned that he had two previous analyses, each lasting three to four years, which terminated because of work commitments in another country, as well as two previous marriages which ended in divorce at his instigation. He had recently remarried for the third time, and this was to be the third analysis. I later learned that he frequently fell in love in a totally idealised way and that when this broke down, the only solution available to him was to cut out the relationship and start afresh. In consequence he was assailed by persecutory guilt as a result of which he felt that he had to give everything he owned to his abandoned wife. His father had died two years previously but he gave no importance to this. I noted that there was a complete blank as to his early years. He had been extraordinarily successful academically and professionally.

On the first day of his analysis, before he lay on the couch, he was acutely anxious and propitiating; he was cautious lest he do anything out of order. He told me that he had been very disturbed when he got into his car that morning to come to his session. He had seen a dark foreigner (he himself is from a country abroad) parking his car in a place which he first called a building site, and later referred to as a demolition site. A huge foreman had rushed over to this man in a manner that was so violent and abusive that he feared that the foreman was actually going to kill this man. My patient had been terrified and the anxiety was still with him. He then told me that when he was filling his car with petrol at the garage close by my house, it had brought back memories of some years ago when a motorist came into a garage and jumped the queue – on that occasion he had feared that anyone who intervened would have killed or been killed, I was acutely aware of his desperate anxiety and of his appeal for help. The fact that I live in a private road which has a large notice stating PRIVATE ROAD RESIDENTS ONLY WHEEL CLAMPS IN USE is obviously significant. After relating all this to me he lay on the couch.

In spite of this overwhelming anxiety, once on the couch he seemed unnervingly calm. He then absolutely repudiated my interpretation that he was feeling anxious in relation to 'parking' himself here, in the analysis. He was very polite, yet there was an implication which became more explicit following that interpretation, that he knew that I would make such transference interpretations, but that as far as he knew there was no evidence to support my interpretation. I tried to use what seemed to me the obvious evidence in the material reported above to validate my interpretation, in the vain hope that I would reach a part of him that would understand. He met this with a complacent rejection. I then felt that any further interpretation which I might make would be 'jumping the queue' and would lead at least to 'litigation' (he is partly in practice as a lawyer). I noted to myself his earlier statement that anyone who intervened whilst queue jumping was in operation was in danger of being killed. My interpretation was not experienced by him as a view which could be linked with another point of view. There could be only one right meaning – his own, and correspondingly he perceived me as unable to consider a view other than my own. He did not live in a world in which someone might bring a new perspective and understanding but one in which there is only one, right point of view, which by necessity excludes all others.

On later reflection my interpretation might have dealt with the nearest to conscious manifestations of the split between his feelings on and off the couch. At the time I was astounded by the split affect – the overwhelming anxiety and the unnerving calm once he was on the couch. Yet he presented such compelling material with such 'obvious' transference implications that I felt impelled to believe that my understanding of his persecutory anxiety in the here and now to be essential. I believed that I could provide meaning and be meaningful to him. I did not realise then that I was 'programmed' to be part of a re-enactment of a critical situation which I shall describe later, i.e. a catastrophic inner situation which needed urgent attention. This enactment bypassed the understanding of underlying crucial emotional issues arising from other parts of himself feeling abandoned. In one way, I was I believe, correct in my interpretation, in another way I was totally out of touch. He too was partly right and in my view totally absented himself from another area.

Some Developments in the Analysis

Quite early on he reported that his wife had returned an unsatisfactorily treated suit to the dry cleaners. He said that he would be terrified to do so, as he would fear the rage of the dry cleaner and believed that he would be 'blackballed' even from the services of other dry cleaners if he complained, though he knew this to be absurd. He came to realise that he believed that any person who offered him faulty service, if challenged, could only take revenge; he had no belief that anyone would listen with concern for his complaint. He then modified this, saying that this did not occur in the institution in which he worked. When I linked this with the analysis and his disagreements with me and feelings of insufficient understanding, he immediately disagreed with me. He said that he felt secure, we had many disagreements, but he always felt that I tried to understand him and he could see my reasoning and my attempts to be fair with him. Although this appeared to be another sign of his compliance, I felt that he was being truthful about his immediate feelings. Once again the split between overwhelming anxiety and absolute calm was striking.

It was around this time that I realised that he had, very soon after starting analysis, recovered and indeed improved his ability to function with interest and enjoyment at work. This suggested that he was also working in the analysis, yet both these improvements remained unacknowledged. He gave all credit for these changes to the support he received from the institution he worked for, even though this support had indeed been available before the breakdown. What became apparent was that for him it was the institution and process of analysis that he found helpful; he emphasised that it was absolutely nothing personal. He dismissed personal contact as irrelevant and unnecessarily complicating, a threat to the institution.

However, on another occasion, the reverse became apparent. He arrived for a session in a very disturbed state and said that he had been disturbed the whole weekend. He gave me an account of a reproach made to him by a junior administrator in his institution; she complained that he disregarded her and did not say good morning to her; she added that 'I know that you are a very senior person, but I am also a human being'. He was terribly upset and asked the woman to see him. It seemed that she had got over this and accepted his apology. He, however, remained tormented, partly believing that he could not have done something so unforgivable and that the whole world would know of this and shun him. This oscillation between massive denial and hateful vengeful annihilation was a regular feature. That is, although he complacently claimed that personal significance was irrelevant, when his annihilation of personal meaning was revealed to him, it constituted the worst of all crimes, and he felt himself at the mercy of a vengeful annihilating superego. Yet in relating this to me he was also turning to me as someone who he hoped would react differently from this superego; he was relieved by the end of the session. Again we see this polarised split between experiences in life and on the couch.

By now there was a long history in the analysis in which any reference to either one of us being personally acknowledged as significant in separation, was treated as an absurdity.

When I drew his attention to this, he would respond – 'You are quite right, it does not mean anything to me'. He believed that he was being friendly; the contemptuous dismissal of me seemed to be miles away from his capacity to be aware of it. It seemed that there was in operation a perverse practice in which, he believed I participated. This involved idealisation of the capacity for dismissal of all thoughts of dependency, a possible repetition of an early experience with his caretakers. The unforgivable crime, in terms of his junior colleague's complaint about him, was that the excluded person was not acknowledged; yet it was impossible for him to acknowledge feeling left out in relation to me. Instead he maintained a separation from feeling, and a denial that I or he were disturbed by issues of separation. Annihilation takes place and it has to be accepted by both sides that it has not happened. (And yet as I will show later, this issue is the fundamental point in his background.)

There were repeated examples of this annihilation of personal significance, with indications that this was both dreadful and that it did not matter. Thus, I had learned that he had been the darling of his grandfather, who especially invited him for weekends, and who out of devotion to the patient, sat through films which he (the grandfather) did not enjoy. When the grandfather died, when the patient was about 12, my patient felt nothing. The family were very upset and cried. He said 'It may be of interest to you Doctor, to know that when I heard of his death I wet my bed on two consecutive nights'. I, of course, was interested, whilst he totally dismissed its significance. He maintained that there was no connection between the grandfather's death, the missing tears and his bed-wetting. He conveyed that he was both subhuman and lacked the capacity to feel love and loss; at the same time he again showed superior contempt in which he was 'above it all'. The underlying phantasy was that he could turn tears into urine, pee on that part of himself that valued a relationship with a helpful, loved person, and excrete the idea that loss was of significance.

Similarly, on another occasion he told me that when his father had died two years before he started analysis with me, he had experienced no feelings of loss though family and friends cried at the funeral. Whilst at this time, he had been aware of his inability to feel, he was dubious of the sincerity of others; only the sorrow of his older sister carried conviction. He felt that the many people who came to comfort the family were all false, yet could not reconcile this with his sister receiving comfort and warmth from the belief that the memory of father was valued and kept alive by so many people. (I shall refer later to the importance of this belief in the authentic, caring relationship between his sister and their father.) Equally, as his analyst, I knew how much our daily contact meant to him, yet this was totally repudiated by him. At best only an impoverished meaning survived until well into the second year of his analysis.

In the beginning I was conducting an analysis in which I had a patient who believed neither in the transference nor in dreams (this notwithstanding the fact that he had had previous analyses). When I referred to this, he presented extraordinarily long detailed dreams. He prefaced this by saying that he knew that dreams were important to analysts; he himself thought that they had no significance. Yet again, I abstracted features of the dream to validate my earlier interpretations, showing him how they demonstrated many features that had arisen in the analysis. This was counter-productive and confirmed his view of his analyst as someone narcissistically obsessed with his own ideas, jumping the queue, and annihilating what was meaningful to him. At that time I had been dominated by the idea that the only way of establishing my significance to him was through persuasion and insistence. This was an important countertransference experience from which I learned a great deal both as regards his early history and how I repeated it. I had the experience and the conviction that there was a child struggling to be included as meaningful, and this very struggle ensured rejection.

Very significant progress was made when he bought to me the problem for him, of his wife's desire to have a baby. He lost his composure, and in agitation said that if there was to be the slightest defect or problem, they should not have a baby. A picture emerged of a continuously demanding, totally unappreciative, inconsolable infant. He seemed to be able to enjoy other parents and their children but this could not be the case for him. He believed and was determined to convince me that he and his wife were absolutely ill equipped for parenthood, and that he alone would have to carry this impossible, unbearable burden. He was not, at this point, seeking understanding or exploration but only my endorsing the affirmation that there must be no baby. This corresponded to the dogmatic way in which he cut out any reference to his own infantile feelings. Working through these problems I began to feel freer and that my hands were less tied. He could now acknowledge that the whole of his infantile life was blocked off and experienced as threatening.

The Disclosure of an Early Infantile Trauma

He had previously insisted that his mother was a totally unimportant figure; when I referred to the mother (or the mother in me, in the transference) his first impulse was to dismiss this as meaningless. Any current contact with her was something of a dutiful formality. Now in the course of such a 'dutiful' long distance telephone conversation he had enquired and learned about his early infancy having told his mother that this was of great importance to him (N.B. to him, not just an interest of mine). It emerged that when he was born, as his mother did not have enough milk, his mother's sister (who had plenty of milk) then breast-fed him. In the first week of his life he developed severe eczema. 'Distinguished' doctors prescribed ointments and his body was covered in bandages; his hands too were covered and tied to stop him scratching. This treatment continued until he was three years old. Mother said that he was wretched. The doctors insisted that they enforce this regime rigorously. Even after the eczema had cleared up his mother said that, if he, for example, touched a marble table, he would experience excruciating pain; he suffered from unbearable hyper-sensitivity. The patient himself was now able to link this (and this was in itself quite an achievement) with the near chronic current hyper-sensitivity of his upper respiratory system. Although this condition was a defect he quickly reminded me that this was also a condition he held in common with a very famous man.

This account threw a good deal of light on my countertransference experience in the analysis. I had indeed felt that my hands were tied just as his had in fact been tied. How does an infant (child) experience human containment which forbade human intervention? Understandably he turned for love to a phantasy of undifferentiated mutual idealisation which pre-existed separateness. His dreams were frequently dominated by cruelty and persecution, increasingly dreams of stripping those who looked after persons in need. These dreams in which the carer was reduced to pretentious nothingness were a frequent theme. For example he brought in one session the following two dreams:

1. His father was alive and treated by a famous doctor (he associated to the famous doctor who looked after his eczema; also an allusion to a pretentious analyst/me). In this dream his father was maltreated and asked my patient to give the doctor a suitable reward. The patient provided a small box of chocolates.

This dream in my view shows his dissociation from himself as the maltreated patient (it is his father who is the patient) and the contempt for the doctor/analyst (provided with a small box of chocolates) who instigated the enquiry into his infantile life. These devices kept at bay the disruptive violence expressed in other dreams, which I shall report later.

2. He came to a session and I was away. A young woman wearing a white coat stood in for me (the implication was 'dressed in her brief authority').

This woman was initially called an assistant, then not really an assistant but a secretary who was not trained to look after patients; not a doctor, not a psychoanalyst; she did not know how to conduct herself.

Although it was me who was absent, I was given the sweetener. Yet there clearly was also a view of me as pretentious, and devoid of any possibility of a meaningful contribution. Yet at this time he was making desperate efforts (in spite of having to travel abroad) to increase his sessions from four to five times a week as he knew he was being transferred abroad and would have to end his analysis earlier than had been planned. The more he realised and now conveyed how much he valued his analysis, the more intensely the devaluation was reiterated in dreams. Love and hate were now coming closer and dangerously together. The earlier extreme splitting which had been employed as a life saver was now becoming less polarised as he came nearer to the unbearableness of ambivalence.

In a dream of this period the entire resources of psychoanalysis were now to be amassed together with the single purpose of saving him, even whilst he wished to show that my efforts were pretentious and meaningless.

For example, in this context he dreamed that:

He was in a place like a barren desert; he felt deprived and desperate. The whole world was 'hotting up' as a result of pollution; there were talks on the radio that the world had neglected to deal with pollution. Listening to the radio he heard that all the countries got together to save his home town (the town where he was born and where his mother and sister live). The town was so hot, some reports said 80 degrees centigrade (this he added, was obviously incompatible with life though this did not cross his mind in the dream). The world had organised a massive fleet of planes carrying liquid to lower the temperature in his home town; it was as if all the planes in the world were assembled for that purpose; they spawned further planes. The sky was full of them. He added as an aside that of course his home town was too far to be reached, that nothing could be done about a temperature of 80 degrees centigrade; he implied that this enterprise of rescue was a gesture, a show rather than a realistic contribution. (He had recently been highly critical of the British Government which had ostentatiously rescued one child from Bosnia while neglecting the holocaust there.)
There were 4 or 5 (he implied useless) guide poles to guide the planes; (he made no conscious association to the 4 or 5 sessions). He was with his wife who said 'let's take one or two of these poles as a souvenir'; he replied that he could not do that, it was quite improper, and in any case they were government property. His wife tried to persuade him to take a

pole. He first firmly resisted, then reluctantly acquiesced. (He told me this in a way that implied that I should take note of his correct stance under pressure.) Then a Range Rover appeared; Prince Charles, the owner of the poles, stepped out. (I knew that he perceived Prince Charles as a derisory figure, someone who tried to maintain a public image but had no idea how to live a personal life.)

As he related this dream it was clear that he was very conscious of the denigration and stripping of my worthwhileness as shown in his depiction of the person who is going to save the world as an empty self-seeker. It did not take him long to realise that he pictured the whole world as failing to look after what should be looked after with consequent terrible retribution – the total destruction of life; pretentious exhibitions of technical caring which were totally inefficacious. The analytic guide poles were on the one hand precious and needed to be saved, and on the other hand reduced to futility. They were anyway the property of someone who did not know how to live but wanted to be in a position of majestic adulation (his view of Prince Charles). The degree of narcissistic omnipotence in which the patient's home town is the selected centre of the world to be rescued and at the same time is the centre of absolutely destructive heated retribution for unwarranted neglect and destruction typifies the impasse of his wish both omnipotently to destroy beyond repair and to be nursed, saved and looked after by everyone. Yet the actual carer, the analyst, is reduced to a hypocritical, denigrated puppet.

The barren emptiness portrayed at the outset is replaced by a total hotting up into manic triumphalism which commands total service whilst all the efforts on the part of the 'world' to repair the damage are rendered futile and hollow, destined to be of no avail. He is heated up to fever pitch to the point of death, that is, psychic barrenness in which no meaningful life can survive. It was not possible in this vicious circle for me to explore how much the barren emptiness was the consequence and how much the instigator of rage.

The extent of the primitive forces at work as revealed in such dreams, now went together with a genuine attempt at working through some of these issues. He was pained to realise what his dreams revealed about his inner world; the abyss between primitive destruction and genuine appreciation. He saw the Prince Charles figure as also alluding to himself, hollow as a drum, unable to live life. At no point did he see himself (or others) as a mixture of some pretension and some real achievement – it was one or the other, both being totally polarised. This excessive split, as I indicated earlier, is central to my theme. Witnessing the capacity of others to engage in an ordinary enjoyable intercourse, created in him unbearable envy which was dealt with by omnipotent triumphalism, as clearly revealed in the dream. He becomes the centre of the world and all awareness of reality is destroyed.

In his early life he had suffered deprivation, pain and wretchedness, feeling that he did not belong, a permanent outsider. (He had been removed from his mother's breast to his aunt's; his whole body eczematous, his hands tied. Presumably the whole 'world' attended to him yet was unable to really attend to his emotional needs.) He became extraordinarily gifted at technical care (his work), winning prize scholarships to major universities outside his country. He was his grandfather's 'Majesty', eventually gained his father's dedicated attention, had many adoring women who were there only to be discarded by him. He had achieved the repeated involvement of analysts. At one time I pictured myself running after him with a spoon, desperate to get acknowledgement, the fate of many women in his life.

I picture this infant, his eczematous skin, hotting up with a rage which is both intensified by his deprivation and restricted so that it cannot be expressed, only screamed out of him. He is driven by this unbearable situation, maddened and tied up, to resort to his omnipotent defences. But once in his omnipotent position his provider now becomes servant to his Majesty. The object's real wish to provide is denied, and all such endeavours are viewed only as technical and pretentious. The failure to provide the understanding for which he craves is met with such hatred that he insists there is no authentic help available; he seems almost to wish to die rather than to admit that he needs help (it has to be found in an 'under the counter' way – getting the guide poles, keeping them and calling them useless souvenirs at the same time). In the analysis he was meticulous in remembering sessions and dreams, was able to link and became interested in the analytic process. The nearer we came to understanding and experiencing personal intimacy the more this faculty broke down. He hated intellectualisation and yet was a master of it.

Later Developments

Gradually, when some integration had developed and he felt that emotional contact was achieved, he ended sessions by saying 'thank you' in a way that was quite genuine. He began to tell me of great improvements in his personal life, as well as a new capacity to develop more human relationships at his work. I had reason to believe that these changes were also noticed by others.

Although at times he looked forward to his sessions he could not acknowledge in a deeply personal way that he wished to see me again or that he had missed me. What he consciously yearned for in absentia was not a creative relationship, which at times he felt he discovered with me, but what he called the experience of 'coming fully alive'; this was always represented by fantasies of love affairs in which there was a vital, lively woman continuously available, adoring and at his service. He could not tolerate any frustration, any delay, without almost immediately replacing the missing object with one that was fantasied as omnipresent and completely fulfilling. Previously he had often told me that in social situations he had to be the perfect host providing total continuous satisfaction; equally when he was a guest the burden fell again totally on him to be the sole perfect provider. He saw no incongruity in these demands. He considered it just that he should be ex-communicated if he failed in either position. This new experience of his reaction to separation from the analysis was the beginning of his recognition that it was he who should be provided with continuous perfect service and at the same time be regarded as the provider. The increasing clarity of this new awareness laid the foundations for a more realistic enquiry about give and take. He had been both the relentless superego and the victim of it.

Yet the obliteration had not been a total psychotic obliteration; he had seemed able both to wipe things out and to keep them encapsulated for later use and yet maintain some internal communication. But the crucial facts of his infancy had been consciously sealed off though, as we see, they governed his life.

In the past he had been convinced that he was totally in touch with unadulterated reality and that I had created a false reality to validate my interpretations; now instead he was disturbingly aware of his own changing reality and he now regarded me as more of a helpmate to deal with this aberration. He increasingly recognised the use of his mind partly to see the world in a realistic way and partly to shape it at the service of his defences and narcissism. The analytic sessions were more fruitful in both his view and mine. He seemed to bring together primitive and more realistic appraisals. From the dreams, however, we could see how unconsciously this situation was misrepresented and then used to maintain his omnipotence.

For example, whilst the analysis appeared to be going comparatively well with the achievement of insight, he produced in one session the following two dreams.

In the first dream

> he is in another part of the world chairing an important international meeting; I am somewhere there, outside the meeting, engaged in writing an academic paper.

As I understand it, I and my work have become of academic interest only, cut off from the place where real life is conducted. But he is capable of achieving integrations on a world scale.

In the second dream

> he is in an exotic place enjoying food; he meets my wife, accidentally knocks over some crockery, whilst I am seen outside on a veranda, completely asocial. He has taken over my position, my capacity to integrate, my wife (he is in an exotic place where he is tasting the special foods) and again I am not there.

These events appear to be flamboyantly obvious, but a new development was his ability now to recognise his own envious and jealous feelings. He feels embarrassed – not regretful. He begins to experience me as a significant person, needed by him. Whereas in the past he had a deep terror of being known, the feeling of being understood was now the basis of some security.

Although from the outset this was known to be a time-limited analysis it was in fact cut even shorter as he was obliged to move abroad at the end of three and a half years. The move was very painful and brought home to him the loss of analytic help, the awareness of separation and of his defences against it. Shortly after hearing about his transfer abroad he dreamed of his father's death and awoke crying and crying. He said 'why should I now be reacting like this to my father's death?' The link to the ending of the analysis had been totally disconnected, but was now easily and speedily recovered in the session.

He told me, somewhat shamefully, that he had not even told close colleagues about his move because he felt that from the moment of telling them he would cease to exist in their minds as a person of any significance. He attributed to them his own ways of dealing with loss and separation, i.e. annihilation of the object and replacement of it with its successor who now becomes the only object of significance, all memory of the original object having been erased. He knew that this was mad and was amenable to understanding that it was he himself who practised this 'killing and cutting out' as a defence against feelings of catastrophic loss. He felt compelled to eradicate the past and get on with the future, and would say to me 'What is the use of dwelling on the past; what good can it possibly do?' There was no internal structure that could support an experience of working through and mourning. I believe this was linked to his experience of his illness being denied by his family. They had behaved as though it never happened. Yet there was a wish that I should maintain contact with our past, and a search for reassurance that he would not be overwhelmed by loss and guilt or the void created to obviate these feelings. This was exemplified by progress in the way he used dreams. Segal (1991) has described the different ways dreams can be used distinguishing between communication and evacuation. This was well illustrated by my patient. His dreams were now less split off from his current feelings in his waking life and more manifestly connected to the work we were doing in the analysis.

His dreams which earlier on had been extremely long, disconnected and were primarily used for evacuation and to disown aspects of himself, were now shorter, coherent and accomplished dream work commensurate with his current reality state. For example he now dreamed

> He was in a town house in his own country (at home). It was small with an extension at the back that at one time accommodated servants (my consulting room is now at the back of the house). Now it is a study room. As the dream continued he took his food downstairs to a private part of the house and there he heard my voice expressing affectionate greeting at the return of a woman friend who had been absent. My wife also appeared in the dream as a sympathetic concerned person.

This was now no dry intellectual study; in the dream he has an affectionate and meaningful father and mother but of course he now has an oedipal problem to face, a new more conscious challenge. His dreams also included references to his wish that I keep him alive in my mind and his attempt to keep me alive. He was now, in reality, in closer contact with his sister and felt fortified by her, sharing with her thoughts about their dead father – a relationship with someone who understood and could share in the loss of a parent/analyst.

He left analysis expressing deep appreciation but with questions in both our minds about the fragility of this improvement. True to form he said 'If ever you are in X and need anything, however trivial, please do not hesitate to get in touch with me. I'll be only too happy to be of service to you' – hinting at the danger of the re-emergence of his apparent obsequiousness, both hiding and revealing the underlying omnipotent superiority. This expressed his wish both genuinely to reciprocate my care and his compulsion to be the perfect provider, with his analyst placed in a position of need.

Discussion

This relatively brief analysis raises many issues. Was the retrieved information about his infancy authentic and does it have any link to 'recovered memory'? How much did this information illuminate or misguide the analytic couple? How useful was this information in the process of working through in the transference and countertransference interaction?

In the light of the massive splitting in this patient, where opposites could not be allowed to come together (so that incongruities in his life had remained unrecognised) the information about his early history helped patient and analyst to extend awareness. I became more in touch with the problem of his inability to believe in personal intimacy (rather than fusion) and the way in which this intimacy was unconsciously both yearned for and feared. This yearning was suffused with grievance which fuelled and was fuelled by envy so that coming alive not only exposed him to frustration and loneliness but to the fear of a catastrophic tragedy in which vengeful hatred would destroy his world. This realisation made sense of his earlier search for intimacy as an undifferentiated union where 'two hearts beat as one', even though he knew that this would end in tragedy when reality would strike home.

This splitting had served a function of promoting survival. Integration was not possible as the only outcome for him was a violent meeting of irreconcilable forces as he so clearly communicated in the first session. Had I been aware of his history earlier I might have given a different emphasis. Not being thus aware enabled me to have the experience in the countertransference of the pain of dependency on an object who negated my meaning. I enacted in vain a demand for understanding knowing that it would be met by a rejection suffused with sadism.

The normal developmental process in which the mother provides a home for the projective identification of the infant and lays the foundation of a faith that the infant is meaningful, was grossly impaired. This absence of an experience in which the infant is enabled to ascribe personal meaning to the mother, resulted not only in the deprivation of mutual meaningfulness, but exacerbated desperate impulses both to find meaning and to vengefully destroy meaning.

The two dreams which followed the information about his history (one in which the famous doctor is rewarded with a small box of chocolates, the other in which the analyst is clearly depicted as an impostor) showed his contemptuous dismissal of caretakers, whose contribution he clearly depicted as meaningless. However as he came to value the analysis more and, for example, radically changed his work schedule to gain an extra session, the conflict between yearning for help and his violent grievances erupted as was clearly depicted in the 'world catastrophe' dream I reported. The vengeance he felt for the way he was treated, the omnipotent reaction and the depiction of desperate efforts to save the world, with the barren consequence, revealed the extent of the impasse. Yet he made use of this realisation to begin the task of re-evaluating his past and later experiences

The question which arises is what it was that enabled him now to embark on this new development? In the past he had employed excessive splitting, keeping the early infantile experience totally sealed off from consciousness. This had presumably included a family conspiracy of silence as though there was a hidden agreement that awareness of those events would be beyond anyone's capacity to manage.

It was only after the understanding of that major dream, which had a considerable impact on him, that he was able more fully to recognise his own violence. This had in the past always been so strenuously repudiated. The experience of an analyst who survived the onslaught and was felt able to perceive and tolerate the violence, without counter-violence, was central. This development had its precursors in the analysis, and in that part of him that had, notwithstanding the splitting, remained able to observe a relationship of love and hate coming together which had ended favourably. I have earlier alluded to the importance to him of the observed passionate relationship between his father and sister. This had played a significant part in his quest to find persons who were authentically truthful and loving, to counteract the pervasive feelings of there being no real concern, only hypocritical imitation.

He had described violent quarrels between them, in which they had insulted each other, smashed plates, slammed doors; he had feared that they would murder each other. But they would always make up the quarrel and were pleased to repair and recreate the lost good relationship. This was a different world which contrasted with his anxieties (evidenced from the very first session) that damage was final, irreparable and devastating and should be put out of mind as quickly as possible. This relationship between father and sister seemed to have served as a model, a live and authentic relationship, which had been kept alive by him despite his insistence that this did not exist.

Later, when he was becoming more integrated and more aware of his aggressive rivalry with me, he dreamed (as I wrote earlier) that he was in an exotic place enjoying food, meeting my wife and accidentally knocking over crockery. He now brings the smashed plates (connected to the rows between father and sister) directly into the oedipal conflict with me.

Whereas in the past the meticulous care he had been given formed the basis for his meticulous academic and professional achievements (in which he had felt well, if not excessively supported by the family) now he had some access to a richer emotional life.

As a postscript I would mention that the patient came to see me very recently, some three years after ending; he greeted me in a warm, affectionate way, expressing much appreciation of his analysis and telling me that I would be pleased to learn of the further changes he had made and that he was now looking forward to the possibilities of he and his wife having a baby. He felt confident in their ability to take care of a baby. Professionally, he was working in the same field and had been asked by the parent body of his organisation to undertake the task of reconstructing and modernising the whole organisation. I thought that whatever degree of omnipotent rivalry might be present, this was an apposite description of the predominantly positive sublimation of our work together.

References

Freud, S. (1917) 'Mourning and Melancholia', *S.E.*, 14, p. 246.
Rosenfeld, H.A. (1971) 'A clinical approach to the psychoanalytic theory of the life and death instincts: an investigation into the aggressive aspects of narcissism', *International Journal of Psycho-Analysis*, 52: 169-78.
Segal, H. (1991) *Dream, Phantasy and Art*. London: Routledge.
Steiner, (1994) *Psychic Retreats*. London: Routledge.

5

Expiation As a Defence

Ruth Riesenberg Malcolm

I wish to deal in this paper with a specific type of defence which organises itself in the analysis into tight, closed, and rigid behaviour that creates an impasse which may make continuation of analysis, as well as termination, impossible. I am referring to those patients who use expiatory behaviour as a form of self-punishment and suffering, avoiding what for them is feared as even greater suffering and danger, namely, their perception of the damaged state of their internal objects – a perception indispensable for any real reparatory work.

The patients I wish to discuss feel their internal world to be populated by damaged or destroyed objects. They are afraid of being responsible for this destruction and feel helpless and hopeless to do anything about it. They have often reached the point in the analysis where some of the persecutory anxiety and schizoid defences have diminished, they appear more integrated, and they have experienced relief. They are on the verge of coming closer to realising how they perceive the state of their loved internal objects. But here they experience a pain of such intensity that it quickly becomes persecutory. They fear this pain to be unendurable and this makes them turn away with hatred from analytical work.

Turning away is achieved by leaning towards masochistic behaviour, which in turn serves the purpose of preventing the emergence of any awareness of their feelings of guilt. Also, being in pain seems to alleviate the guilt. They feel they are making expiation – that they are being incessantly punished for what they believe is the damage they have done. This punishment takes the place of what instead should be reparation, that is, restoration of internal objects that have been attacked in fantasy. Through reparation, a modification of the internal world is achieved; it becomes more benign and therefore growth can take place.

In most analyses we get momentary or temporary expiatory reactions. But in this paper I am describing situations in which the whole analysis is being turned by the patient into a continual failure for the analyst, with its aim to produce punishment. In 'Mourning and Melancholia', Freud (1917) described a similar type of condition and he pointed to the links with introjection and identification. In 'The Ego and the Id' (1923) he referred to the polarity of life and death instincts, and suggested that the negative therapeutic reaction was related to the death instinct.

In her classic paper about the negative therapeutic reaction, Joan Riviere (1936) used the recent discovery by Melanie Klein of the depressive position, and she emphasised the role of manic defences, particularly omnipotence and omnipotent denial of psychic reality. Riviere especially pointed to the need to recognise the positive feelings of the patient, suggesting that what the patient most fears is that the process of improvement would lead to suicide or disintegration.

Klein, in her paper 'Envy and Gratitude' (1954), added to Riviere's formulations. The hatred aroused by admiration and appreciation of the analyst's good capacities (and the internal objects represented by him) increases the tendency toward a negative therapeutic reaction and, in turn, increases the unconscious feelings of guilt. In the same paper Klein also spoke of the problem created by 'the stifling of feelings of love and corresponding intensification of hate, because it is less painful than to bear the guilt arising from the combination of love, guilt and hate'.

I have referred specifically to some points in the literature on negative therapeutic reaction, since I consider them to be closely connected with the type of analytic problem I am trying to describe. Nevertheless, I believe that there are some differences between the patients that react with a negative therapeutic reaction and those in whom expiation predominates. These latter patients react to the analysis with something that could be thought of as their motto: 'no change provides safety from pain and disaster'. Organising their whole behaviour in the analysis so as to create a static situation that consists of their own suffering and misery plus the analyst's immobilisation, they feel that this static condition encapsulates or puts their dread within limits; it contains it in such a way that they do not have to actually face it. Bion (1963) refers to a phenomenon that is similar to what I am trying to describe here. In what he calls *reverse perspective*, the patient also tries to achieve a static condition, but does it secretly. The immobilisation of expiation is not a secret. He clings to a situation of non-analysis in a setting that is nominally analysis, and feels that this state of affairs should last for life. The patient's awareness of being able to produce the halt in the analysis also brings feelings of triumph, often linked with sexual excitation. This erotic satisfaction contributes, in part, to the perpetuation of this type of behaviour. The patient believes that he avoids or denies his helplessness through keeping things as they are. He projects his helpless self into the analyst, and also his own potential for perceiving guilt. Through the use of those projective identification mechanisms, he not only feels that he has rid himself of those feelings and problems, but also avoids the responsibility; for now the analyst is the guilty one.

These dynamics, the belief in having succeeded in ridding himself of the dread of madness or death, together with the sexual gratification, both masochistic as well as sadistic, place this problem close to the area of perversion. Here I think it worth remembering Glover's paper 'The relation of perversion formation to reality sense' (1933), in which he describes sexual perversions as defences used by the patient against psychosis.

Along with the patient's fear of harbouring damaging and accusing objects, the patient also has a relation to an idealised omnipotent primary object. The emergence in the analysis of contact with this ideal object (experienced in the transference as the analyst), and the patient's own good feeling toward the ideal object, sometimes permits a breach in the otherwise steel-like enclosure, and proper analytic work can take place. But the patient will generally react to this achievement in two ways. On the one hand he will feel pleased, sometimes relieved, and will be more generous. This encouragement makes the patient feel that the analyst has been sufficiently reassured, so that the patient feels he has removed any danger of the analysis coming to an end. On the other hand, progress fosters the patient's hatred because he feels quickly exposed to those very conflicts that he is trying to avoid, and thus he will reinforce his attacks on the analyst's competence. From the analyst's point of view, this type of encapsulation and the occasional breakthrough that permits a more hopeful view of the patient's loving and constructive capacities, undoubtedly complicates the whole range of countertransference responses.

The combination of these factors makes the analysis go in circles. The patient's interest is to prevent it from progressing, since the so-called 'analysis' is perceived by him as confining his problems to the analytic sessions without further consequence. The analyst feels that he can neither help the patient nor terminate the analysis, because the patient's expiatory behaviour presents a continuous danger of suicide or disintegration. Both analyst and patient are locked in a difficult, even impossible, situation. Should termination be contemplated, *both* patient and analyst are faced with a sense of absolute irreparability.

Clinical Presentation

Mr K came to analysis primarily with the desire to become an analyst, but also to get some help with his problems, the most important of which he felt to be indecisiveness. He described himself as a 'compulsive doubter' and 'the most successful failure'. In his first interview he reported a profuse symptomatology. His aspirations were bizarre and he was intensely arrogant and incoherent. He was also obviously in considerable pain. He showed some warmth as well as a fine sense of humour. It was very difficult for him to leave the interview.

Previous diagnostic consultations with different psychiatrists had resulted in apparently different diagnoses, all along lines of psychosis or borderline conditions. A previous analysis had lasted three years, and turned into a three-times-a-week psychotherapy. The analyst ended abruptly in a way that seemed to me to be very traumatic, but Mr K spoke of this with both glee and triumph.

Mr K was the only son of what appeared to be a very disturbed family. He described his mother as an 'extremely good person': 'She always wanted the best for me'. From the beginning he repeated that she had used influence to get him into exclusive schools and other circles. But she worked full-time, and actually took no personal care of him because of what appeared to be excessive anxiety. Mr K nonetheless always spoke of her with reverence. The little time she spent with him was spoken of as not merely good, but nearly perfect. He used to say this in a flat voice with no feeling. He also said that she worried very much about him, fearing that he did not grow, put on sufficient weight as a baby, or was not pretty enough. In the preliminary interview he communicated something that would recur frequently in the analysis, namely, that he had never told her that he loved her and that she died before he thought of doing so, when he was seventeen.

The father emerged from the patient's description as hard and indifferent, not sharing much of his life with the family. The parents were separated for approximately two years when the patient was two years old. Mr K's father had died before the analysis began.

During Mr K's first year of life he was looked after by a quick succession of nurses. Then a permanent nanny arrived, who stayed until he grew up.

Despite many problems in infancy and childhood, Mr K finished school, studied at a university, and obtained a degree and a professional qualification. He emigrated to Australia partly because he could not get along with his father and also because his mother used to tell him that this would be 'the best place in the world to live'. In Sydney lived his mother's sister of whom he said he was very fond. He went to Melbourne and there suffered his first major breakdown and had to return to England. He spoke of his coming back in many ways. He stressed how besieged he was by doubts about returning but also said that he needed 'to make it up with father before it was too late'.

But when he returned, trouble with his father started again and during a very violent row, his father told him to go to his room. He stayed there, literally, doing nothing for a year. Finally, he made himself leave the room, studied his father's craft, making jewellery, and in spite of disliking it, worked at it part-time.

Phase 1: The Psychotic Transference

I would like to divide the account of his analysis into three phases. In the first, the patient was highly disturbed. He often had flights of ideas, made many puns, constantly mocked everything, and he sometimes hallucinated. In the first week of his analysis he spoke of a dream and an incident with his father, both of which would bear considerable importance in his treatment. The dream occurred during the night before his first analytic session with me.

> He was in a village inside a ditch, and had to climb up to get to freedom. He had in his hand a kind of miner's pick, but when he proceeded to make his way up, an enormous amount of rocks, earth and all kinds of heavy things fell on his head. To his surprise, the first association that came into his mind was a very thin girl whom he knew. At that time she was about to leave London to go south.

As can be imagined, my interpretations of this material were very tentative. They were related to his fear of what the analysis might do to him or what he might do in it. I also mentioned that he might be worried about my strength: would I have to run away? (My accent as well as my appearance suggest that I might be native to a southern Latin country.)

The incident he told me about had occurred when he was ten years old, and he related it with a mixture of worry, satisfaction, and hatred. His father asked him to go and buy cigars for him. The patient provocatively asked 'Where?' His father, irritated, said 'Stanmore', the location of the jewellery workshop, some forty-five minutes from home. Mr K did exactly that, going to Stanmore and coming back some two hours later. He spontaneously volunteered an explanation. He said that he had always been very passive and wanted to be told what to do. He said this in a strange, very flat voice, sneering at the same time. He also said that the actual place where his father wanted him to go was in fact opposite their home, but the patient did not like the place. He thought it was frequented by prostitutes and he felt ill at ease there. He said that he had always hoped that his parents or grown-ups would guess how he felt.

At the time, I noted how immensely heavy Mr K felt and how despairingly he experienced the approach of the analytic task. I also noted that I felt uncomfortable about the way he spoke of the incident with his father. I wondered how much he would use sadistic sexual acting out. From the beginning of the analysis Mr K reacted very intensely to weekend separations. After the first analytic holiday he came back in a severe state of depression.

In this phase, as in the following one, he often communicated concretely through action rather than verbally. He used to wear ragged clothes, especially a pair of old trousers, full of holes, as a way of showing me how impoverished, miserable, and broken he felt. He usually came in a long coat, several sizes too large for him, that had belonged to his father, and he kept emphasising that it was 'his dead father's coat'. (When we started the treatment, his father had been dead for several years.) In the sessions, he moved around the room, sat on the floor, or stood immobile near the door. He often felt that I suffered from delusions.

In this first phase material emerged that threw light on his early infancy. We learned about his severe feeding problems. He often reacted to my interpretations by turning them into a meaningless mash which he would let ooze out in the form of fragmented sentences, words, and mere sounds. I learned in what way disintegrative processes were in operation and also that he had to get rid of its products very quickly. In response to my interpretation of this material, he told me that he had been informed that he had suffered a severe diarrhoea during most of his first year of life or a bit longer, and that this drove his mother frantic. We then were able to link his behaviour in the transference to experiences in his early infancy.

In the transference, I stood for all kinds of part or whole objects. There emerged with great clarity a division of me as a very powerful mother (or breast), that could give him anything if I so wished, and as a nurse, I could make him normal – be his analyst or make him an analyst, that is, somehow let him become me. Or else I was felt to be rigid, just giving him interpretations, keeping set times, a harsh nurse determined to feed and clean him. Occasionally I was a more intermediate figure: not too bright, quite insensitive, just wanting him 'to adjust', the nanny who wanted him to be a well-behaved child.

In a paternal transference, he perceived me as stronger and more aggressive, ready to criticise. He had to win me to his side, conquer me, or fight me. All this was done in a highly erotised and teasing way; and it felt very homosexual.

In spite of the severity of pathology, genuine progress took place. Mr K's relation to me changed and his material became more coherent. He started again to report dreams (which had stopped for quite some time); he developed a passion for them because their analysis brought him great relief, as well as understanding. He stopped hallucinating.

Phase Two: Extreme Control

Together with these positive changes, new aspects began to appear in the sessions; it is those which I refer to as the second phase. Mr K began to control me more and more. He produced two or three repetitive themes with the aim of proving that I could do nothing; at the same time, he really expected me to provide an answer that would solve his problems at a stroke. For example, he would ask me a question, generally practical and referring to an actual situation in his everyday life – for instance, whether he should post a letter. I was ordered to answer in one of four ways: 'Yes', 'No', 'I don't know', or 'I cannot answer because it is against the psychoanalytic technique'. It was irrelevant what I interpreted or if I actually answered as he demanded, because when I did so he proceeded to find a flaw in the answer. Whatever I said, or if I said nothing, it always drove him to recite the alphabet again and again, sometimes for the duration of several sessions.

I initially tried to deal with this development as ordinary material to be interpreted in the whole of the transference context. Since I could not reach him this way, I would begin my intervention with 'I don't know', and try to explain the reason why I was in no position of knowing, and how the problem seemed to go further than the realm of the question and answer. I added that he might be very determined to get an 'answer' from me but that I thought he also might perceive my interpretation differently. He would answer that all that was irrelevant since I had spoiled 'his orders' by going beyond the sentence 'I don't know'. He would ask why could I not just say 'I don't know', or why could I not say 'that it was against the technique'. My attempts to remind him that he knew (from his own statements in previous sessions) that the technique was no more than a part of a process would be interrupted.

At some point I managed to get across (and I wish to remind the reader that most of the time he was monotonously reciting the alphabet) that his questioning me, together with his need to make me obey orders, suggested other questions that might feel upsetting to him, which probably felt too painful and were related to the way he was treating me. Therefore, by turning me into a mechanical answering machine he believed he could avoid those potential upsets. Sometimes his whole manner would show that he was touched by my words. But the hatred of having been touched and therefore losing successful control would increase his anxiety, driving him to intensify the monotonous recitations.

On the occasions in which I would just say 'I don't know', he might speak about something else, but then promptly repeat the original question. He would say he was not sure if my response was 'the answer' or just a 'catch'. I tried as far as I could to point out both his controlling behaviour and also the fears I thought were underlying this control. I remarked that the dread he might be experiencing made him fear that everything was a trick. I also attempted to link his fear of guilt with the sadistic satisfaction he was getting from his behaviour, and how this in turn made it more difficult for him to get out of his psychological state.

Another theme, his complaints about his life and work, also applied to the analysis. Mr K would say in a very tormented way: 'I drill holes and fill them up with silver; that is all I do'. He drilled into all my attempts to interpret and filled the sessions with repetitions of the alphabet. In turn, I often felt as if my mind were a sieve. I could remember very little from the sessions, but was preoccupied with what was going on in them. My mind was not functioning during sessions, but it did not wander. The reason for this, I believe, is that he had a powerful hold on me, probably through a minute type of projective identification. I remember an occasion on which I was very preoccupied by a problem of my own, and it came fleetingly into my mind during a session. Mr K stopped saying whatever he was saying, and sat up in a panic.

This behaviour lasted for many months. I think that due to all the effort, very slowly one could see a mixed response. He tried to harden himself even more against my interpretations. He even brought a tape recorder into the sessions with the explanation that he had no memory.

With this new development, I felt very uncomfortable. But I accepted the machine at first, because I knew that should I refuse it the likelihood was that I would not be able to enforce my refusal. I also thought that if I succeeded, it was very probable that Mr K would perceive it as an increased success: I would be doing what he had been demanding all the time: 'giving direct orders'. With him, I kept my instructions to an absolute minimum; the analysis took place in the consulting room at set times and the door would be closed. With the rest of his actions, I tried to deal with them through analytic interpretations.

I felt that the tape recorder, moreover, showed two main things: his behaviour was leaving him without a memory, that is, without a mind, and that he also had a desire to remember. I oriented my interpretations from this second aspect. I emphasised the pains and difficulties arising from his continually trying to put out of his mind almost everything by questioning and, even more, monotonous chanting of the alphabet. There was some positive explicit acknowledgement from him in the midst of his acting in.

Together with the appearance of the recorder there was, at first, increased bizarre behaviour, I think probably as a response to how he perceived my feelings. But in spite of some mockery, his desire to remember was taking first priority, to the point of his genuinely stating 'I did not want to lose what you were saying'. His recitations diminished and an increase of violence in his associations came to the fore.

Once, upon entering the room, he looked with horror at the couch, stood very still, and asked me if there was a four-poster bed where the couch used to be. He said that he saw it. I will try to summarise the content of many weeks of work on this issue. The main associative theme was prostitution and a pub called 'The Blind Beggar'. During this time, news reports were following a trial that was taking place. A criminal gang that used to terrorise the East End of London was being tried. It had just come to light that the gang's means for obtaining their objectives was torture. The gang operated from the Blind Beggar pub.

As I have mentioned before, Mr K's main mode of communication was through actions or tone of voice. At this point I felt, from the way he was speaking, that something very dangerous was going on, and for the first time in this analysis I actually became frightened for my safety. I used my fears as an orientation of where to put the emphasis in the interpretations. (I also took some practical measures of protection, such as having a nurse in the flat who would come should I ring an electric bell near my chair.) The content of the interpretations pointed mainly towards the operation of a torturing gang inside himself, directed against both me and the self who wanted 'to remember', to learn, and to know so that he could feel better. This cruelty in him was so terrifying that he felt we had to submit to it to prevent further and worse consequences. I linked it to blindness – so as not to get insight, not to know, since the guilt of seeing what was going on was threatening the most intense pain. In that way, he felt better to be a beggar, to get nothing, rather than the awareness of this awful sight. I also, very slowly, emphasised that now, in spite of the torturing terror, he was more able to look at what was going on in his mind. He could now bring it more into the open, speak about it and, though half-heartedly, try to remember the meaning it had for him. The half-heartedness came from the question: Who was remembering? Himself? Or a machine without responsibility?

While working in this area, my fears progressively diminished and I dispensed with the nurse. Mr K made repetitive attempts to increase and harden his control, while at the same time his cruelty towards me became more vicious. Nevertheless, I felt that he could keep an increasingly continuous contact, mainly through interpretations that he could take and which allowed for an alternation between cruelty and genuine understanding. This allowed him to attempt to control the cruel behaviour and he tried to work with me. Those attempts, however slight and short-lasting, had a real constructive quality, and marked changes occurred in the sessions. The recitation disappeared almost totally. He began again to bring dreams and work at them. Glimpses of changes in his external life emerged. He seemed less isolated, spoke about people, and resumed his original profession part-time (which he liked better than jewellery and which he had stopped practising because of excessive anxiety). His relation to a girlfriend seemed to become less bizarre.

It seems to me that many factors had played a part in producing those modifications (I am speaking of work done over a period of years). The decrease of the need of such a sadistic control was partly due to his perceiving me as a strong analyst and thus able to contain his 'horrors' without being completely overwhelmed by his anxieties and therefore more able to present them back to him (reintrojection) in a modified way (Bion, 1962). He experienced gratitude and a desire to make good, which in turn brought new incentives towards further understanding which, in small quantities, could be used by him.

In other words, through the increase of introjective processes a more benign relationship was setting in which allowed for the possibility of structural modifications. His superego (internal objects and an internal analyst) became less cruel and punitive. His ego as well became stronger and therefore much less in need of resorting to extreme modes of defence. The following vignette might bring a clearer feeling of what I am trying to say. In one session, he said rather angrily that I was like one of the nurses he had as a baby: 'She must have been a brutal beast'. He had been told that she even sat him on top of a wardrobe to get him to eat. I said that this could be taken as beastly, but that I also wondered if he might not be saying, however angry it made him, that he recognised my efforts as like that of the nurses in childhood: not letting him starve or go hungry. I added that we might have been trying to get the baby in him to take something in, since food, mental food, is important for life and growth. He was moved by this and felt thankful. He said 'I have to give it to you, you do try and if something does not work you try something else, in spite of me being so beastly to you. Either you are not too frightened or you still go on in spite or whatever'.

This improvement in the analysis lasted for some time, after which I began again to feel myself progressively more limited in my thinking (this time it felt differently – more oppressive) and in my capacity to reach him with my interpretations. A new repetitive theme started to establish itself in the material. He began to produce endless variations of one sentence: 'I made a mistake'; 'A mistake happened'; 'It is all because of a mistake'. The mistake to which he referred was that he came back to England instead of staying in the ideal place, Australia. As one may imagine, I tried to deal with this material from many angles – all to no avail; and then I realised that I was totally stuck. We were in what I call the third phase.

Phase Three: Stagnation

With phase three, Mr K had reached the most difficult point in his analysis, for along with the improvement, feelings of guilt became paramount. However difficult the previous two phases were, for the patient this last one appeared to be insurmountable.

The themes were very repetitive, circling mainly around the same contents. For example, Mr K would walk into the room, not looking at me. Once on the couch, instead of speaking directly, he would say something like 'Shall I talk to you or not?' Or he would recite a long rigmarole, always the same, which amounted to asking me whether he should write for an application to the Institute of Psycho-Analysis.

In spite of the immense repetitiveness of these sentences, the feeling they conveyed to me was far from being always the same. Sometimes it seemed to be a plea to give him a helping hand that would allow him to start. Sometimes he did accept the help and began to speak directly about the issues that were in his mind. But of course this did not always happen. There were very subtle nuances in how he said things that did allow me to sense different things.

On other occasions, he sounded more excited and whatever I said then was discarded. If I said nothing, this was taken as a hostile provocation or as proof that I had been put out of action. When I did speak, be it an interpretation or a description, Mr K would meet it with great contempt. He would tear it to pieces and the 'mistake' was brought to the fore, generally in a very plaintive, monotonous, nasal tone, immediately followed by a superior attitude to prove that, since the mistake took place twenty years ago, it was of no use for either of us to try to understand anything at all.

During this period, Mr K suffered intensely, but according to him, I also had to suffer, so he had to 'drill it into me'. One of his fears was that otherwise I would not know how he felt. He again resorted to the use of massive projective methods and concrete behaviour. Also he believed that this was sexually stimulating for me, that it must be exciting, 'kept me on my toes', particularly if he could believe that he was hurting me. (My main feelings were very painful, and a couple of times I did actually get a very short-lasting, sharp stomach pain. He perceived the whole situation as turning into a flirtation, a sexual game.)

He also had the conviction that I had the power to put things right, but, of course, not through analysis. For him this meant putting the clock back twenty years, and turning him into an analyst. He believed firmly that a word of mine would make him accepted into the Institute of Psycho-Analysis. He felt that I was very cruel not to do this, and it stimulated him to further cruelty to prove how useless I was.

Through very careful listening to his way of talking, rather than its content, since what he said was usually very much the same, I could sense a possibility of making contact with his anxiety. It is possible that I must have felt him more receptive and myself less tied up. I tried to do something that I had done before, to produce just descriptive summaries. Generally, as also in most of my interpretations, I would start from his state of pain, his desire to draw me into attacking him, and therefore become actively 'the punisher'.

On other occasions I could sense from the way he was speaking that he was actually aware of thinking something else – or was preoccupied by something – and I would try to point this out to him. He would show surprise at my noticing it, and would allow associations to flow and would listen to interpretations. For example, one day he was reciting his litany: 'Oh! that terrible mistake, why, why did I do it?' I felt that in spite of his usual monotonous voice, which he called 'tuned-down-flat', he was agitated. I also felt myself becoming more alert. I ventured a comment in which in fact I said that I thought that he was agitated, and that it might be that this monotonous litany might also refer to something else. He was startled, and started speaking about having been very worried because of something he had said to a colleague that he thought might have been very unkind.

This instance, as well as some others, allowed for some analytic work to take place. He could then take in some understanding about his unkindness to me – originally the nurse – and the fear it gave him to look at it. We also worked on the fact that the 'not looking' made him feel that he lived *ad aeternum* in 'a mistake'. He became more depressed, his whole demeanour changed, and he would appear very worried. During these times he shrank from any interpretation of his positive qualities as a person, since this seemed to increase feelings of guilt as well as fears about his ability to sustain his good qualities. For example, if I would refer to his concern about someone at work, he would react with a mixture of pleasure and fear – fear that would often lead him to mock me and himself or try to prove the contrary. 'Me, doing something good! You must suffer from excessive imagination!'

I believe that 'the mistake' was also an attempt at encapsulation, though of course not exclusively that. But a mistake, just one, however badly it made him feel, also allowed him not to have to look at many things, 'many so-called mistakes', in his behaviour towards his objects. Furthermore, the mistake consisted in leaving the land felt ideal by his mother. He had behaved very nastily to many people in Australia; he did break down; he 'was expelled from Paradise'.

At other times, Mr K was in a more receptive and sad frame of mind. He would puzzle about why he behaved towards me as he did. He would question whether he was a pervert. These questions were sometimes mocking, but more often they were serious and concerned. On occasion my interpretations were oriented toward how much he worried about this. In spite of trying to laugh it off or reassure himself that I was a masochist and that was the reason I put up with him, he had doubts. He felt that his behaviour was not only hard on me but incomprehensible to him, that just to say that he was 'a pervert' did not mean much, and that he needed to look into this cruel, gruelling behaviour that he called 'perversion'. I sometimes also pointed out to him how much he wanted me to call him a pervert; the word would then acquire a moralistic meaning and he could feel me accusing and punishing him. In other words, through projective identification, I would be the punisher, and he would avoid his own anxieties. When I managed to get this across to him (and he did not feel I was punishing him), he experienced intense pain that drove him into panic, which in turn prompted him to intensify the cruelty of his behaviour by a total grinding of my interpretations, rendering everything – that is, what I had said and his own understanding – meaningless.

If he did not succeed in this, and my words had some impact on him, he would force himself to sleep in the session in order to cut off all contact. He would also force himself into sleep when he came with the desire to tell me something he felt important. This felt too dangerous to him.

One of my greatest difficulties with this patient was to avoid being too repetitive, and to try to be alert to any minimal change in his way of speaking or in the way he inflected words that could be used for either a new approach or for a new way of addressing him.

I also felt more and more under internal pressure. The idea of the scarcity of time kept creeping into my mind. I often found myself thinking that 'I had to do something', or it would be 'too late'. 'I had to think of something.' I think that I might have contributed to his own fears by 'trying too hard', until I realised and became clearer about the projections into me of feelings of irreparability. I could then orient my interpretations, starting from my feelings of pressure and his feelings about time passing. (He spoke often about this, but I do not think that my reactions were due to actual, external reality.) I became more watchful so as not to overinterpret, and tried to increase my containment of the situation for longer stretches of time. During the whole analysis I had let him talk or act at length, but I felt at this point, maybe not sufficiently, that he needed even a longer time. In spite of his intense suffering he needed me to wait and wait, and only then to interpret. This projective identification was aimed at testing whether I could endure him without going out of my mind. But it required a careful balance. If waiting was perceived just 'a fraction too long', it was also proof that my mind was out of action.

In spite of all these difficulties, he managed to convey something that made me feel slightly hopeful, and also very sorry for him. After a period in which the balance between a total paralysis of the analysis and some more sensitive understanding was tipped a bit towards the latter,

Mr K became very depressed. His external life deteriorated. He complained often that he could not cope any longer and he interrupted analysis for some time. Guilt became very prominent. He warned me about the possibility of his stopping, several weeks before he actually did so. I think that the idea might have been in his mind for a longer time, considering the intense pressure I kept experiencing of 'having to do something'.

He approached the subject of stopping the analysis in two ways. First, he said he had no money, that he was spending more than he was earning, and he could not afford it. Of course, I think what he could not afford were his depressive feelings. Second, he just had to stop. His explanations came out so muddled that I cannot reproduce them here. His language was almost incomprehensible. He moved as someone attacked by most intense pains that could not be described in words. He acted as if under a tormenting force that dragged him away from me. He could not 'stand coming to analysis'. I think I was then felt by him as an internal analyst (externally he could be more warm and friendly to me) pulling him to the struggles between love and hate, life or death. He maintained that he could not stand this, that he had more to lose than to gain, much like a baby who, as soon as it allows itself to be fed, gets bouts of colic and diarrhoea. Mostly those feelings were projected into me – hence, the conviction that stopping would bring relief and possibly freedom.

He broke away from analysis, kept telephone contact with me, and eventually asked to come back. During the interruption, he had pulled himself together. He had started working full-time. He felt triumphant and hypomanic. He felt that he had cured himself in the same way, whatever that was, that he had got himself out of the room in his father's house. He also reacted triumphantly to my taking him back.

Why did he come back? And why did I take him back? It soon appeared that the flight into so-called 'health' couldn't be maintained and that he was in panicky fear of collapsing, of becoming very depressed and of falling to pieces. He acknowledged only some of this when he asked to be taken back, but he did agree that now he was not coming for analytical training but as a patient in need of treatment.

My reasons for taking him back into analysis were mixed. I was aware of the dangers of not doing so. But I think it was predominantly his capacity to stimulate hope in me about making some fundamental change, as well as the projection into me of the need to do something. Looking back, I think I felt trapped in the situation which I described at the beginning of this paper, which is what makes it impossible to terminate an analysis. I think that I, as well as he, found it impossible to face the idea that he might be beyond repair. Though I was doubtful about the wisdom of taking him back, I discussed it with a colleague; I think I was more inclined to cling to hope.

Some Further Background Details of Mr K

I would like for a moment to consider some aspects of what I have been saying about this patient.

I think Mr K had achieved a relationship to an object, a whole object, but this relationship was never firmly established and developed. It is my opinion that his tendency to idealisation when he was an infant was expressed in multiple associations and reactions to interpretations. 'Mother was extraordinarily good', 'kind to a superhuman degree, she rushed from her death bed to take a gift to a charitable society'. In the analysis, when something really did satisfy him he used to have a very strange, blissful smile or he would praise an interpretation or my capacity of making it, in a way that had no basis at all, either in what I did or said. For instance, when I once made an ordinary, pedestrian interpretation, not new, but to which he had not listened before, he said, with a kind of radiance, 'You are Shakespeare!'

The idealisation, a normal factor in any infant development, was probably accentuated in Mr K by constitutional weakness. The split was between the very bad mother (breast) and the extremely good mother as expressed in his analytic material. This split was much stronger than in ordinary patients and, I think, probably was also reinforced by his mother. Not only could she not contain his anxieties but projected her own anxieties into the child and needed continuous reassurance from him. She was always worried that he might not be well and dragged him from doctor to doctor. This was to the intense annoyance of the patient's father, who found no sign of things going badly and contrary to the view of the paediatricians. He had also been told that, when little, as soon as he and mother were together, he laughed and made all kinds of 'cute things for her'. Whatever he told me about what went on at home with his mother, some of which sounded either harsh or bizarre, there was never a note of criticism. Also, there was never any praise for a nurse or nanny.

In the analysis, with me as the ideal mother, he invested me with omnipotent powers. I could turn him into someone else: a very successful analyst. I think that as an ideal mother I was to get him right inside me, through his being fused with me, becoming me. I was the mother who got him into 'exclusive places' (the only child). He also felt compelled to tell me very often how intelligent I was, or how my interpretations sounded poetic – often when these remarks were completely alien to the general feelings he was having at the moment.

The deep splitting between the ideal mother and the bad persecuting nurses, and the difficulty of bringing those aspects closer together was, I think, also influenced by another factor. It is my impression that as soon as he would get close to mother physically he became very excited. This excitement seems to have spoilt the contact, confusing him as to what was the quality of the object he was in contact with.

This confusion was seen in ample transference manifestations; deeply hostile as well as friendly actions were so intermingled by excitement, that it was often impossible to discern what was going on. It required a very lengthy, patient, and minute observation while holding the situation.

This extreme idealisation of his mother made it much more difficult for him to work through guilt. Since his perception of mother was of a perfect object, and therefore any damage to it made the guilt enormous. And he felt helpless to repair the damage unless he himself was omnipotently perfect.

The conjunction of these factors made his capacity to bear pain, which was probably constitutionally limited, almost non-existent. Therefore, guilt was perceived as a horrible experience and had to be avoided at all costs.

Finally, the paralysing of the analyst, together with the avoidance of guilt, seemed to express a passive early experience of an inadequate external object. His reliving this in the analysis appeared to have the aim of communicating the experience of a passive helpless mother; but, at the same time this communication was turned into something pleasurable in itself. This erotisation, which in the analysis appears perverse, may have stemmed from an early experience, probably perceived as very confusing by the child, in which he felt that if he could act sexually he would enliven the object and make it less anxious. I think this explains, at least partially, his conviction that somewhere there was some pleasure for me in all this.

Once Mr K was back in analysis, after the short period at the beginning in which he was hypomanic, he made a genuine effort to work in the analytic sessions. But soon he relapsed into the ways I have previously described, this time in a worse form. He sometimes reported dreams literally in only the last one or two minutes of the session. They were often of concern to me and contained elements indicating potential suicidal danger. When I tried to refer to them the following day, Mr K would not let me talk and would go to sleep, etc.

Two dreams were the last ones he reported before a complete paralysis took over. Unusually early in the session, looking very depressed, he reported the following.

> I was walking through a very dangerous path, probably mined, full of barbed wire. It was surrounded by police, just standing there. It was in Connaught Square and I felt that if I managed to walk through, I would be free.

This last remark was painfully sincere. Then his tone changed. He seemed to force himself to mock me. He said 'Well, we lived right next to that place. Nanny used to take me there for walks. All right, come on. What can you make out of this?'

I pointed out that perhaps Connaught Square might also refer to something else. To my surprise, this silenced him and after some thought he reported that when watching TV the previous night, he saw a program about the siege in Connaught Square. The IRA were holding a couple as prisoners in a flat. He added that in the dream, he did reach the other side and was safe. He looked very subdued.

My interpretation was that he seemed to be suffering from a severe conflict that had been with him since childhood. He knew he had to go through something very difficult to reach safety and real freedom. These difficulties felt horrible to him, both internally and externally. If he attempted to walk, he feared that he would be torn into pieces (the wire), this probably having to do with separation from his objects, both me and the original one. His insides would explode like the mines. It is striking that no helping hand existed and so he surrendered to an aspect of himself that ordered him to freeze everything, including the transactions between the analytical couple. There is a connection here with the imprisoned couple in the flat.

The patient was extremely quiet. After a moment he went on to say that he had 'a bit of a dream' following the previous one and with the same theme. He described it as follows

> I want to reach freedom and safety. To do so I have to dig a tunnel and go through it. While I am digging it, I see the gravel and rubbish piling up into a terrible mess that makes me feel that I will never be able to clear it up.

He had awakened abruptly at 3 a.m., feeling extremely depressed. After this description he complained about becoming increasingly slow in whatever he did. He could not function.

This session was drawing to an end. I tried in my interpretation to link the two dreams. I said that if he functioned in the analysis and he used me properly, he would see such a mess that he feels hopeless to put it right. But that he also felt me to be helpless, as somebody held in a siege, paralysed like the policemen, paralysed by his behaviour in the previous sessions. It is his perception of me as being helpless that added to his hopelessness. If I was allowed to help him, and also, if he was aware of the mess, then both of us would have to clean it up. He felt very badly about it – so badly that he became panic-stricken with the fear that he would not be able to bear it. So he had to stop everything, even the dream by waking himself. He left the session looking extremely depressed. The next session he slept the entire time. I tried to reach him by reminding him of the similarity between the dream he told last session and the one he dreamed at the very beginning of his analysis. He jerked, opened his eyes, and went back to sleep. I don't know how much he had listened, but I think that he heard something.

I waited. I tried now to link both dreams to the anecdote he had told me in his first session (both of those memories from that first session came suddenly and spontaneously into my mind). I pointed out that his fears of the consequences of his provocative and stubborn behaviour made him not only feel awful but also made him perceive me as an internal father, impotent to help him with the gravel. So he had to shut himself off by going to sleep. Again he jerked, opened his eyes, closed them, and started a rhythmical breathing so as to induce sleep.

He slept the entire time as well as in many subsequent sessions. It was impossible to re-establish any contact with him until he could completely resume the old pattern of repetitiveness which made the analysis static.

I want to end this clinical presentation with these dreams, which I consider to be very revealing, because they express his hopelessness as well as his determination to paralyse and maintain the siege. As a result of his own determined effort, he returned to his usual mode of stultifying behaviour. I was totally paralysed, while he suffered, complained, and demanded, as an immediate omnipotent cure, that I should turn him into an analyst.

The analysis went on in this manner for many months. It became progressively impossible to reach him. By now I was faced with a decision. Was it advisable to go on in a situation in which the analyst is no more than a guardian-nursemaid or a perverse sexual partner? This, of course, in addition to its uselessness, increases the patient's guilt. Or does the analyst have to take steps to end the treatment, facing the consequences this may have?

I finally decided in favour of ending the analysis. I waited for some time before actually telling him, in order to see how this decision might influence my work with the patient. I felt freer, but things did not change at all.

I gave the patient slightly less than a term of notice (approximately two months, a considerably shorter time than is my usual practice). I decided on this shorter time to give him a chance to do some work toward termination but also to not to make the termination time so distant that my announcement might appear to him as more threat than fact. Also, in my wording of the announcement I did not leave open the possibility of continuing with me.

Discussion

I want to limit my discussion to four main points extracted from the vast range of problems that a patient such as the one I have spoken about presents: (a) specific difficulties in the analysis with this type of patient; (b) some comments on the problem of expiation; (c) the impingement of this type of psychopathology on the analyst's emotional responses; and (d) some considerations about technique.

Early in the paper I mentioned that from the patient's point of view, stopping the analysis carries serious danger of suicide or disintegration. As many authors have already pointed out, this danger underlies many of the problems that bring about a negative therapeutic reaction. I think that the specificity of suicidal danger in an expiatory defensive constellation consists in the patient's carrying his expiation to the last consequences, for himself as well as for his internal objects. These patients will reach the climax of suffering by dying, which is what they fear most. The other specific consequence of this syndrome is that patients will disintegrate when they do not have an external container, in which to encapsulate, *ad aeternum*, their problems. Those problems, when having to be held back, drive them to defensive fragmentation, which may end in a permanent state of disintegration.

Riviere (1936) said that what the patient fears most, should he make contact with his inner world, is suicide and disintegration. It is my belief that for the type of patient presented, it is the analyst who actually fears those two possible outcomes much more than the patient himself. This fear in the analyst, conscious or unconscious, creates a state of anxiety closely linked with guilt, which I think in turn is stimulated and increased by the patient's projective identifications.

My experience, both in directly treating patients as well as in supervising colleagues, has shown me that the sense of failure, the incapacity to effect reparation with these patients, makes the analyst react in an anxious way. I do not mean acute anxiety, which is easier to detect and therefore to attempt to understand, but a kind of diffuse anxious state that expresses itself in a 'pressure to help to alleviate pain'. This may explain the sometimes overextended length of the treatment, when the same analyst, with other patients, could have concluded either to interrupt or to suggest a change of analyst, with more clarity of judgement. He will experience the usual pain and difficulty but without the agonising feeling that 'one has to go on' or that the patient cannot be abandoned. I have seen the same type of response in analysts with very different personalities, as well as some with different theoretical backgrounds.

In dealing with this kind of problem, and especially in treating Mr K, I often wondered whether it was something specific to the patient's mental make-up or whether it was due to something shared by the analysts that treat those patients. I do not think I can answer this question with any accuracy. My observations make me think that the reactions of the analyst are mainly caused by the specific problems of the patients, especially their use of projective identification. But I am also led to believe, with not enough evidence at present to substantiate it, that there may be a common factor in the therapists' reactions, probably related to their personal modes of dealing with depressive anxieties.

In relation to the psychopathology of 'expiation', one aspect deserves emphasis. I have spoken of this expiatory defence as a perverse organisation, or even a perversion. I have mentioned the frequent use of erotised and excited manifestations in the analytic relationship. What I have not spoken about is my belief that what is sexualised is 'the pain' itself. I do not mean the suffering, which I think can be more easily deduced from the expiatory behaviour and is a common character in masochistic pathology. What I mean is that the perception of any contact – physical at first in early infancy and mental later on – is perceived as painful. This pain is immediately sexualised. This sexualisation of very elemental units of pain serves to facilitate a pervasive expanding of generalised erotisation. How does this take place? I do not think I can give an answer at this point. I can only state that in my observation it does take place and it could be of interest to find out why.

During the exposition of Mr K's analysis and of the problems that arose in it, I mentioned many examples of countertransference reactions, feelings, or acting out. In explaining the difficulties in terminating such an analysis, I expanded on some specific countertransference responses. I want to end the subject of countertransference by mentioning what I think was my greatest block in perception. This was not Mr K's sadomasochistic behaviour, but the fact just mentioned, namely, that most early contacts were perceived as painful, and that this pain was immediately turned into sexual experience. When I finally could see this, my first reaction was a mixture of dismay and disgust. A colleague from another country, whom I supervised in the treatment of a similar patient, also went through the same difficulties and reactions. I wonder if this could express such a twist in the relation to the object that the destructive impulses – whether reactional or primary – are so intense that they becomes almost indigestible for the analyst.

While I realise that my comments on this last point are not sufficiently illustrated in the material I presented, they are very difficult to describe in an account of sessions. However speculative, they are worth consideration.

Conclusion

I would like to finish with a brief reference to my technique. The patient's behaviour in the consulting room at most times was very bizarre, to say the least. Still, I consider that what was going on was a classical analysis, inasmuch as my method did not deviate from the ordinary analytic technique. The patient behaved as did some psychotics and children that I have had in analysis. I took his behaviour as analytic communications which I tried to understand and interpret in the framework of the transference relationship. My interpretations, whenever possible, were guided by what I felt to be the predominant anxiety. I did not interpret symbolic contents, but I worded my interpretations in such a way as to deal with what I believed to be preconscious expressions of his defences, as well as of contents which I hoped would lead to my understanding of genetic explanations.

The idea of introducing what Eissler (1953) has called parameters crossed my mind several times. I concluded that such an action would only be a way of bypassing what I felt most difficult to bear. In reflecting on the patient's possible reaction to the introduction of parameters, I became convinced that they would not only be unhelpful but actually damaging, since they might make him perceive my behaviour as an

5. Expiation As a Defence

expression of my having been destroyed analytically. I also thought that it could increase his anxiety as well as his feelings of triumph. In fact, I hold the view that extra-analytic interventions are in no case of any use. If there is any chance of helping a patient it is only by analysing (Riesenberg, 1971).

As to whether patients with expiatory behaviour can be helped, I do not have an answer. From my limited experience, I would suggest that better results are possible in patients whose expiatory organisation is not so impenetrable that it both prevents the analysis from continuing and also makes the analyst feel that it cannot be terminated.

References

Bion, W. (1963) 'Elements of Psycho-Analysis', in W. Bion (1977), *Seven Servants*, New York, Jason Aronson.
Eissler, K.R. (1953) 'The effect of the structure of the ego on psychoanalytic technique', *Journal of the American Psychoanalytic Association*, 1: 4-143.
Freud, S. (1917) 'Mourning and Melancholia', *S.E.*, 14: 237-58.
—— (1923) 'The Ego and the Id', *S.E.*, 19: 3-59.
Glover, E. (1933) 'The relation of perversion formation to the development of reality sense', *International Journal of Psycho-Analysis*, 14: 486-504.
Klein, M. (1954) 'Envy and Gratitude', in *Envy and Gratitude and Other Works*, pp. 176-235. London: Hogarth Press, (1957).
Riesenberg, R. (1971) 'Die Werke von Melanie Klein', in *Die Psychologie des 20. Jahrhunderts*, Zurich: Kindler Verlag.
Riviere, J. (1936) 'A Contribution to the Analysis of the Negative Therapeutic Reaction', *International Journal of Psycho-Analysis*, 17: 304-20.
Segal, H. (1967) 'The curative factors of psychoanalysis', *International Journal of Psycho-Analysis*, 43: 212-17.
—— 'Melanie Klein's technique', *Psycho-Analytic Forum*, 2: 197-211.

6

On Remembering, Repeating and Working Through

Joseph Sandler and Anne-Marie Sandler

A useful starting point for this contribution is Freud's paper on 'Re-membering, repeating and working-through' (1914), as it provides a good basis for assessing some of the changes which have taken place in psychoanalytic technique in the years that followed.

In his paper Freud points out that, at the start, when he was using hypnosis, the aim of the work was to get the patient to remember, and through remembering, to abreact, to release the pent-up emotions that were associated with the forgotten memories. Later, when he had given up hypnosis, 'The task became one of discovering from the patient's free associations what he failed to remember'.

Freud went on to say that the analytic technique had become one in which the analyst did not try to focus on specific problems, but allowed himself to study whatever was present at the time on the surface of the patient's mind, i.e. the patient's associations. Interpretation is used mainly to show the patient his resistances to the analytic work; after the resistances have been dealt with, the patient 'often relates the forgotten situations and connections without any difficulty'. Here we can see how much importance Freud placed on the *recovery* of repressed memories from the patient's early life. In fact, in his paper Freud says quite explicitly that the aim of the analytic technique is, from one point of view, to fill in gaps in memory, and from another to overcome resis-tances due to repression; but of course the aim of overcoming resistances to analysis was itself directed at allowing repressed memories to be recovered. Even if the real memories are not accessible, relatively innocuous memories from childhood – screen memories – will be revealing. He says: 'Not only *some* but *all* of what is essential from childhood has been retained in these memories. It is simply a question of knowing how to extract out of the them by analysis. They represent the forgotten years of childhood as adequately as the manifest content of a dream represents the dream-thoughts'.

Further, Freud refers in this paper to a special class of experiences for which no memory can be recovered. These are experiences which occurred in very early childhood and were not understood at the time but were *subsequently* understood and interpreted. The knowledge of these early experiences, he says, comes through dreams. He goes on to discuss repetition, which is seen in a particular group of patients who do not remember anything of what has been forgotten and repressed, but who *act it out*. 'He reproduces it not as a memory but as an action; he *repeats* it without, of course, knowing that he is repeating it.' Transference is seen by Freud at this point only as a piece of repetition of the forgotten past. The greater the patient's resistance, the more extensively will acting out (repetition) replace remembering. It is necessary for the analyst to work on the acting out, which represents the illness brought, not as an event of the past, but as a present-day force. The analyst has to try to get the acting out into the mental sphere. Here the attachment to the analyst through transference is important. To limit acting out the patient is asked not to make any important decisions affecting his life during the time of treatment.

Freud then introduces the notion of the transference-neurosis, which is the analytically desirable replacement for the patient's ordinary neurosis. It can be regarded as an artificial illness which enters the transference and is consequently accessible to the analyst's intervention. This then leads 'along the familiar paths to the awakenings of the memories, which appear without difficulty, as it were, after the resistance has been overcome'.

Working through relates to the overcoming of the patient's resistance. It is not enough to point out the resistance, Freud says, but one has to *work through* it; and it really is work, for the analyst and patient have repeatedly to explore the same themes in different contexts, because resistances have a very persistent quality. Freud makes the famous statement 'this working through of the resistances may in practice turn out to be an arduous task for the subject of the analysis and a trial of patience for the analyst'.

It is of some interest that Freud placed so much emphasis on remembering in 1914, but the topic was not fully considered until much later, in his paper 'Constructions in Analysis' (1937a). As we shall presently be referring to this topic from a particular present-day perspective, we should like to say about Freud's views as he was approaching the end of his analytic lifetime.

In this 1937 paper Freud considers the sort of material brought by the patient and repetition in the transference and says 'What we are in search of is a picture of the patient's forgotten years that shall be alike trustworthy and in all essential respects complete'. But he goes on to say that it is the analyst's task 'to make out what has been forgotten from the traces which it has left behind or, more correctly, to *construct* it'. Here we should note that for Freud, 'construction' and 'reconstruction' of the past were synonymous. He relates the work of construction or reconstruction to the work of excavation undertaken by the archaeologist, but the analyst is at an advantage, says Freud, because he is dealing with something not destroyed but is still alive in the present – 'All of the essentials are preserved; even things that seem completely forgotten are present somehow and somewhere, and have merely been buried and made inaccessible to the subject'.

It is very clear that Freud saw construction as a way of getting the significant repressed memories of the patient to the surface. In construction, unlike interpretation, 'one lays before the subject of the analysis a piece of his early history that he has forgotten'; and he adds that if the patient is given an incorrect reconstruction, no harm is done because the patient is untouched by it. Freud took the view that in a successful analysis one gets to the correct construction, that is, to a memory of what actually happened, to what he called the *historical truth*.

Spence (1982) contrasted historical truth with *narrative truth*. He pointed out that the truth of an interpretation or reconstruction can never really be known. In his view the analyst constructs a 'history' which satisfies certain aesthetic and pragmatic criteria, and interprets within a narrative tradition in which what counts is coherence, consistency, and the persuasive power of the narrative. This approach was also taken by Roy Schafer. For both these authors, narrative truth, in place of historical truth, represents a way of explaining the past and provides apparent certainty in place of knowledge which is unreachable.

There can be little doubt that this is a view which is important and relevant to our topic today, one which is consistent with the modern view of the nature of history. Freud had an essentially different approach, having certainly been influenced by nineteenth-century historians such as Ranke, who took the view that the task of the historian was simply to show 'how it really was'. As the British historian E.H. Carr put it in 1961, 'The empirical theory of knowledge presupposes a complete separation between subject and object. Facts, like sense impressions, [are said to] impinge on the observer from outside and are independent of his consciousness. The process of reception is [regarded as] passive: having received the data, he then acts on them'. But in contrast (to the empirical theory), the 'so-called basic facts ... are the raw materials of the historian rather than of history itself ... The necessity to establish these basic facts rests not with any quality in the facts themselves, but on an *a priori* decision of the historian'. However, from the point of view of the psychoanalyst, just as for the historian, it must be said that the past is not merely convenient fiction. We shall touch on the issue of narrative truth again later.

It is striking that in the psychoanalytic literature, even in recent years, a certain degree of confusion between *remembering* on the one hand and *reconstructing* on the other has persisted. But it now seems that, as far as memories are concerned, we need to make a number of further distinctions not only between memories and reconstructions, but also between what actually happened, what the child's experience was of what happened, the phantasy component in the memory, the memory as modified during the process of development, the memory as changed by defences and as reported by the patient in the analysis.

At this point we should like to suggest that it is useful, and indeed necessary, to make a distinction between *construction* and *reconstruction*, and shall not use the two terms synonymously. Construction can be taken to relate to the creation by the analyst of meaningful insights into the patient's *current* inner world. From this point of view we not only reconstruct the past, but as analysts we construct, for example, the current internal object relationships of the patient, we construct the mechanisms of defence being used by the patient, and so on. Such constructions are not memories allowed to come to the surface through appropriate interpretation. They are interpretations of significant and relevant aspects of the structure and function of the patient's mind. We make such constructions in order to increase the patient's insight and to expand his knowledge of himself and his inner world, to help him make a model of his mind, so to speak.

So, for example, the patient may bring experiences of being frightened of policemen. He tells the analyst he is frightened of his bank manager. He is frightened of colleagues at work and, of course, he is frightened of the analyst. In the course of our analytic work we show the patient how there seems to be a threatening part of himself, or a frightening internal figure which is externalised on to others, and in the transference onto the person of the analyst. We *construct* from all the phantasies which have the same theme, particularly those which point to an underlying, unconscious transference phantasy, the notion of a specific internal object and the relationship to that object. We would emphasise that this is not in itself a reconstruction of a memory (although it may evoke reports of memories). It is a *new* formulation which allows the patient to have meaningful insight into how he or she functions in the present. What we construct does not necessarily reflect exactly the structure of the child's mind as it was in infancy because of the process of development which has occurred since the early months and years.

For example, there might have been, in the course of the person's developing phantasy life, projection of aspects of the self onto the phantasy figures who were internalised as an aspect of the individual's internal objects. We know that the superego introjects, the internal objects which we regard as constituting the superego, will contain a great deal of the projected aggression of the child, with the result, as Freud has shown us, that the introjects may be very frightening although the parents may have been tolerant, benign and kind people. One can give many examples of constructions which show the patient how he or she functions. We think of one of our patients, a non-psychotic, normally neurotic person, who whenever she brings associations, dreams or clear transference material, is clearly making abundant use of the mechanism of projection. It has been very important during the course of the analysis that she has become aware of the fact that this is a habitual mechanism of hers; and a great deal of working through has been involved. She is now very aware of this propensity in herself and this awareness has been of great help to her. A construction – or in other words, a structure of insight – has been created.

As far as *reconstruction* is concerned, we can occasionally get confirmatory memories from the early past through a reconstruction of the past offered to the patient, but we do not believe that this occurs all that often. What does frequently happen is that memories are evoked from after the age of four or five, from the latency years, and we have as analysts the habit of taking the memories of childhood from that age and dating them earlier, pushing them back as if they were early experiences. In fact, the memories from before the first years, before the repression barrier has been constructed, with the resulting infantile amnesia, are very fragmentary and scattered. We think that valid or veridical memories from the first few years, including memories of early phantasies, are far fewer than is generally believed, in terms of being able to be recalled with any precision. What are more frequently brought are memories which have been reorganised or early events told to the patient by relatives. The main aim of reconstruction, as we see it, is the *anchoring* in the past of the present picture of the patient and the constructions about how the patient currently functions, so that the present, particularly the present as shown in the transference, can eventually be formulated in terms of the past. This provides a *temporal dimension to the patient's view of himself.* The main aim is not to discover what went on in the past, to release repressed material (although such release may be a sign that the analysis is progressing), but rather to construct a relevant picture of aspects of the past in order to discover and understand better the *present* psychic structure and conflicts of the patient. It could be said that we need to have a picture of the past in order to understand the present for the benefit of the patient's future.

In our view it is technically most appropriate for any reconstructions of the past made by the analyst to be aimed at throwing light on the present, on the here-and-now of the session, to *reinforce* the understanding of the present rather than to be part of a psycho-archaeological expedition. Such reconstructions have to fit the patient's current experience both cognitively and affectively, but should correspond as much as possible to the patient's history and memories: yet they should not slavishly correspond to them. As we have indicated, we hardly ever know the truth of what actually went on in very early childhood, apart from whatever knowledge the patient has received second-hand – even then we cannot be sure of the truth. Ideally we would like to get as close as possible to the child's early experiences and phantasies, but this is not that easy. So in our work of construction and reconstruction, we do not simply try to recreate past experiences or to retrieve memories. In order to make the present understandable we may, for example, attribute motives to the parents in our reconstruction of the past. Thus we might have to show the patient, on the basis of the transference-countertransference experience, that the parents were unconsciously perceived as having been very sadistic, in spite of the fact that what the patient remembers is the kindness of the parents. The transference may indicate something quite different.

It is appropriate to add a reminder here of a point made by Freud in 'Analysis Terminable and Interminable' (1937b), that there is a great deal in the past which cannot be reached. Dormant conflicts are not accessible. We can only really be concerned with what becomes active in the present, in particular that which is revealed in the analysis of the transference. We have the impression that as analysts we tend to underestimate the extent of the unreachable part of the patient, and this makes may of us conduct our analyses for far too long. There is an advertisement for a particular beer which is said to reach the parts that other beers cannot reach, and some people feel like that about their brand of analysis. But it is clear that there are always parts that analysis cannot reach.

It is necessary to say a word about development and the repetition compulsion, which is, of course, a descriptive concept, not an explanatory one. We know repetition seems to dominate the lives of our patients; at the same time we have to take into account the fact that there is not an exact parallel between the present and the past, as we often tend to assume. Unconscious conflicts in the present do not necessarily reflect the identical conflicts in the past. We could say that the present is not isomorphic with the past. It is not symmetrical with the past. During development such things as change of function occur. To take a simple example, let us imagine that someone has developed a special interest in playing the piano stimulated by a childhood need to deflect wishes to masturbate because of conflict over such wishes. The piano playing becomes a sublimation of the masturbation. Later this person, by now a musician, develops a piano playing inhibition. To see this inhibition as a conflict over masturbation in the present may be quite wrong; it may reflect a conflict over competing with the father, over death wishes to the father, for example – the piano playing may have undergone a change of function.

Returning to reconstruction, we should like to put forward a view which derives from our clinical work. We have made a distinction between what we have called the 'past unconscious', and the 'present unconscious' (Sandler and Sandler, 1983, 1984, 1987, 1994). We know that at about the age of four or five a great many developmental changes occur, culminating in the creation of a major repression barrier leading to the infantile amnesia. We take the view that we can never get direct access later to what lies behind the repression barrier. It remains as *past unconscious*, the developmental product of those first few years, which can be seen as a major psychoanalytic conceptual basis for understanding the experiences and behaviour of the patient in the present. In a sense we can refer to the past unconscious as 'the child within'. On the other hand, the notion of the *present unconscious* can be regarded as the area of the mind containing the current preoccupations and the unconscious wishful phantasies which represent the immediate counterparts of those infantile reactions which we attribute to and locate in the past unconscious. This present unconscious is much more accessible to us, but not entire accessible, because of the existence of a barrier between the present unconscious and consciousness, a barrier which corresponds to what Freud (1900) referred to as the 'second censorship'

134

between the preconscious and perceptual-conscious systems of the topographical theory.

From the point of view of motivation, the concept of the past unconscious differs significantly from that of the dynamic unconscious in a number of ways. In the first place, it is not simply composed of drive-invested wishes. The child of five is not simply and only a drive-dominated animal; nor is the child of one, two, three or four. There are also impulses which have a peremptory quality, a force behind them, impulses, for example, to defend oneself – to deny or repress or project, or to have megalomanic phantasies which restore self-esteem, impulses to relate to an object in a particular way, and so on. So, in our view it is unwarranted instinctual drive reductionism to regard all impulses attributed to the past unconscious as instinctual wishes or as drive derivatives. If we look at children of five or younger we see that their motivation is very complicated. For example, anxiety is as strong a motivating force as the drives. It is useful to conceptualise the processes *in the present* as involving, to a large degree, *parallels* to these childhood reactions and tendencies, parallel impulses which disrupt the equilibrium of the present unconscious. These adult impulses are a reflection of tendencies which once were consciousness-syntonic. But because these adult impulses (modelled on those of childhood) cause conflict they are not acceptable to the adult's consciousness, and evoke defensive activity. An adult here-and-now version of the conflict occurs and our work in analysis is first to analyse such current conflict, particularly as it arises in the transference. In this connext Hanna Segal has remarked (1981) that 'in the phantasy world of the analysand, the most important figure is the person of the analyst', but clearly this does not imply that every interpretation has to be a direct translation of what the analysand says into transference terms, even though a transference element may always be present in the patient's communications.

It is appropriate to ask at this point what the relation is of the past unconscious to the present unconscious of the older child or adult. In previous formulations the view was taken that impulses and wishes pass in some way from the past unconscious and enter the present unconscious. They then have to be dealt with there because they may be no longer appropriate, and therefore disruptive. We would now put it somewhat differently.

What happens is that the initial unconscious reactions or impulses of the individual are formed *as if* the person were a particular five-year-old child; and these reactions then have to be dealt with in the present

135

unconscious *by the person of the present*. The child within acts as a *template*, a structuring organisation, so to speak, for the immediate here-and-now unconscious strivings and responses of the older individual. We might even be tempted to call it a psychic agency, a macrostructure. The impulse or wish that arises in the depths of the present unconscious is not one that has been passed through a censorship from the child within – the censoring, if one wants to call it that, takes place throughout the present unconscious, with a final censorship or defensive transformation – Freud's second censorship – before admission to conscious awareness. The unconscious wish arising in the present unconscious is modelled on the inner child's wishes, *but the objects involved are objects of the present*. Let me put it another way by reference to the example we quoted previously. If an unconscious hostile wish towards the analyst arises in a patient's present unconscious, then it is not a death wish towards the father displaced on to the analyst in the transference. Rather, it is a hostile impulse arising in the here-and-now towards the analyst, quite possibly *modelled on* the inner child's hostile wishes towards the father.

However, we are not only dealing with impulses, wishes or phantasies in this context. Reactions to promptings and demands of the external world can be regarded as being initially responded to *as if* by the child within, but to the extent that the responses in the present, modelled on the past unconscious, are trial actions found to be inappropriate to the present or threatening to the individual's equilibrium, they will be defended against and censored, either inhibited or allowed to proceed to action and conscious experience in a modified form. All of this occurs, of course, extremely quickly (Sandler and Sandler, 1994).

When we speak of reconstruction (as opposed to construction) we are talking about what we relate to the past unconscious. In our reconstruction we make use of metaphors, even if we may not realise that our descriptions of what we assume to have gone on in the past (persisting in the past unconscious of the patient) are metaphorical. We build a picture of what we believe went on and goes on in the child's mind and our different analytic points of view give us different metaphors. So we may talk about splitting the breast into good and bad, or of separation-individuation, depending on what our point of view is. But our reconstructions have to fit, intellectually and emotionally, and therefore our reconstructions cannot be at random. They should, as far as possible, fit what we reconstruct of the past, with what the patient recalls, and need to be related to what is going on in the present.[1]

If we approach this topic from the point of view of phantasy formation and transformation, it could be said that unconscious phantasies arise in the depths of the present unconscious, and that they are transformed in their passage towards the surface. They can be regarded as phantasies in the here-and-now, not arising from the past unconscious, but modelled on it, *given shape by the past*. Thus transference phantasies are, in this model, products of the present unconscious, but to varying extent given shape by relevant processes ('procedures') in the past unconscious.

It is a curious fact that, whatever our psychoanalytic orientation, the metaphors relating to our view of infantile functioning are often used to describe here-and-now processes in the present unconscious as if what occurs in the present is simply something early being repeated. These metaphors relating to early infancy can be regarded as code names for what is going on in the present; they are constructions disguised as reconstructions. When one reads the French literature, for example, one cannot fail to be struck how the important phantasies behind the repression barrier can be very different from those which are used in the frames of reference currently employed in Britain. For instance, in France clinical analytic references to the primal scene abound. In Britain it is relatively rare, we think, to reconstruct primal scenes as real experiences (as opposed to phantasies). We do not think that the experience occurs less frequently (although perhaps our bedroom arrangements are slightly different!) but rather that primal scenery is not as much in the mind of the analyst, and as a result the same material may be seen in a different way. What is important is that a good reconstruction will have a resonance with what actually happened, and with what has been experienced in the transference. Although we do not know what actually happened in the subjective experience of the young infant, the reconstruction should have that feeling of being a good fit.

What we wanted to show in this paper is how, for many analysts nowadays, there has been a substantial shift of emphasis away from remembering as an aim of the analytic work. Further, not everything that the patient brings should be considered to be a repetition of the past. Acting out – a better translation of the German *agieren* is 'enactment' (Sandler, Holder and Dare, 1970) – is not necessarily a form of remembering, and transference is not necessarily a simple repetition of an early object relationship. This shift of emphasis is technically important, because it focuses attention on the value of *constructions* about the patient of the present as well as of reconstructions of the person of the past, of the child within. Such constructions, particularly those based on the analysis of the transference as well as reconstructions of the past, of what we might call the 'reconstructed' unconscious – of course contribute to the structures of insight which enable the patient to become more tolerant of unconscious wishes and feelings which had been defended against, and which had brought about problems in his life.

Notes

1. We have to attribute secondary process functioning to the past unconscious as well as primary process; but it is, of course, a fallacy to assume that thinking can be divided simply into primary and secondary thought processes. There are many levels of secondary process functioning, and the small child of five with pre-operational thinking will have very different secondary process thinking from the child of, say, seven or eight who, when remembering something from the past will, in the process of remembering, reorganise that past. We want to stress that the concept of the past unconscious does not correspond precisely to the system Unconscious of the topographical theory or to the id of the structural theory. It is very important for the analyst to take these various levels of secondary process into account. Many psychotic phenomena, for example, do not reflect primary process, but rather primitive secondary process functioning.

References

Carr, E.H. (1961) *What is History?* Harmondsworth: Pelican Books.
Freud, S. (1900) 'The Interpretation of Dreams', *S. E.*, 4-5.
—— (1914) 'Remembering, Repeating and Working-Through', *S. E.*, 12.
—— (1937a) 'Constructions in Analysis', *S. E.*, 23.
—— (1937b) 'Analysis Terminable and Interminable', *S. E.*, 23.
Sandler, J. and Sandler, A.-M. (1983) 'The "Second Censorship", the "Three-Box Model" and some technical implications', *International Journal of Psycho-Analysis*, 64: 413-25.
—— (1984) 'The past unconscious, the present unconscious and interpretation of the transference', *Psychoanalytic Inquiry*, 4: 367-99.
—— (1987) 'The past unconscious, the present unconscious and the vicissitudes of guilt', *International Journal of Psycho-Analysis*, 68: 331-41.
—— (1994) 'The past unconscious and the present unconscious: a contribution to a technical frame of reference', *The Psychoanalytic Study of the Child*, 49: 278-92.
Sandler, J.; Holder, A. and Dare, C. (1970) 'Basic psychoanalytic concepts: VI. Acting out', *British Journal of Psychiatry*, 117: 329-34.
Segal, H. (1981) 'Melanie Klein's Technique', in *The Work of Hanna Segal: A Kleinian Approach to Clinical Practice*, New York: Jason Aronson.
Spence, D.P. (1982) *Narrative Truth and Historical Truth*, New York: Norton.

Blocked Introjection/Blocked Incorporation

Roy Schafer

The first time I heard 'blocked introjection' used in a clinical discussion was at a meeting at which Hanna Segal was the featured discussant. It was a meeting of the psychotherapy staff of the Yale University Health Services, some time around 1970. Segal used 'blocked introjection' masterfully to pull together some basic but disparate issues in a case presentation. In the years since then I have frequently witnessed her (or read her) doing equivalently impressive things of that sort, so much so that she has established herself for me as a model of acute clinical listening and shrewd interpretation. But it is just with the idea of blocked introjection that I shall be concerned here.

The sources of this idea can be traced all the way back, first to Freud (1905, 1917) and perhaps especially to Karl Abraham (1916, 1921) in their essays on the oral phase and depression and, subsequently, to the firm psychoanalytic foundation provided by Melanie Klein. I believe, however, that all of us have experienced moments when a known, interesting, but until then perhaps only subsidiary idea was transformed into an important instrument of understanding by someone's felicitous use of it. One thing we mean when we say of an idea that 'it clicked into place' is that we have successfully introjected an aspect of a mind at work in such a way as to change a piece of learned content into an essential tool for coping with consequential issues. Still, at that moment the process is not yet complete, for further transformation will take place as one becomes more familiar with that new tool, extends its uses by adapting it to unexpected problems, and defines its limits. This process of mastery may be unending. So it has been for me with 'blocked introjection'.

In this essay, in order to detail my present understanding of blocked introjection, I shall explain my preferring to call this unconscious phantasy 'blocked incorporation', then cover some of the complex theoretical and clinical issues that I have encountered in interpreting it, and go on to give some brief clinical illustrations of my uses of those interpretations.

'Introjection' belongs to a family of terms that includes identification and incorporation, the three of them falling under the general heading of internalisation (Schafer, 1968). Of these, only incorporation refers directly to the unconscious phantasy of taking into the bodily self something perceived as existing outside that self. Elsewhere (1972) I have argued that the entire language of internalisation is founded on the phantasy of incorporation. That incorporation phantasy concretises self, mind, learning, restraint of action, and other such ideas, changing each into a substance existing in, or a physical process taking place in, spaces with more or less distinct and confining boundaries. The language of internalisation organises mental events in the terms of a spatial *metaphor* or *story line*. Mental events are not things that travel in space as things may in the everyday physical world. The spatial metaphor of internalisation actualises an unconscious phantasy.

Usually, the concrete incorporation phantasy is cast in oral terms: sucking, biting, chewing, swallowing, gastro-intestinal events, and the like. Although the phantasy can be cast in anal, visual, tactile, and other bodily terms, it is not easily divested entirely of its oral origins; we see that this is so in those familiar interpretations that point out the use of the anus, vagina, eyes, or ears as mouths.

Certainly, the literature developed by Klein and her followers contains an abundance of references to incorporation. In general, the physical, bodily, substantial prototypes of modes of object relatedness have figured prominently in that literature. It has seemed to me, therefore, that the most apt term for the process in question is *blocked incorporation*, not *blocked introjection*. The concept implies the mouth (or its equivalent) shut tight against intruding objects. 'Blocked' itself adds to the concreteness of the idea. For this reason I depart a bit from the more common Kleinian usage: blocked introjection.

I have also argued (1968) that a place should be made in our thinking for 'primary process presences', more simply 'presences'. These presences are the influential phantasy figures who are not necessarily located within the bodily self and whose psychic existence does not necessarily raise questions about how they got to be 'inside'. They may be imagined anywhere: alongside one, lurking in the shadows, and so forth; they may not be placed in any definite space, simply having the attributes of thereness, as in 'I felt your presence even though I know you were not in the room'. The presence may be a whole person or only a voice or a pair of eyes or ears or a skeleton rattling in the closet. *Presences*, in my sense of the term, are part of common experience, and they do not qualify as malignant hallucinatory events; rather, they may best be regarded as daydream fragments so vivid as to feel real without compromising seriously the person's current reality testing. They need not be 'borderline' phenomena. Perhaps 'momentary dreamlike states' comes close to it.

Incorporation may culminate in the experience, conscious or otherwise, of an introject or, if carried further, in an identification whereby the subject takes on its characteristics as his or her own. Here, I shall not be concerned with end points; rather, my concern is with incorporation as a mediating and enabling process.

In certain contexts the phantasy of blocked incorporation may be primarily defensive of the self; for example, in the exclusion from the bodily self of bad objects or substances and their less concrete manifestations in bad ideas or feelings. The phantasy may, however, be in the service of protecting the object; for example, not damaging it by destructively cannibalising it or immersing it in the badness or destructiveness of one's internal world. The reverse of both these dynamics may also be indicated at times, that is, one may be blocking the incorporation of another's goodness in order to avoid destabilising a defensive posture of one's own that features an anhedonic, bitter, or dead mode of function ('not getting my hopes up' or 'not letting my defences down'). Similarly, one may be using blocked incorporation as an instrument of war in object relations by employing it as a punitive refusal of invasive or controlling caretaking and reparative efforts (spurning embraces or 'food that's good for you'). On account of this reversibility, the meaning of blocked incorporation must be arrived at only in specific, individualised clinical contexts.

When blocked incorporation figures importantly in the analysand's emotional life, it will control his or her development of transference and attempted manipulations of countertransference. To avoid confusion in this realm, it will be well to remind ourselves of a major fact of life in psychic reality: the coexistence of more than one unconscious phantasy pertaining to the same relationships and issues and the inevitable contradictions that are tolerated unconsciously. We have been introduced to examples of this fact of life in many places in Freud's work and, with regard to internalisation, in Abraham's as well. For present purposes, consider the case of the analysand who refuses food owing to the phantasised cannibalistic significance of eating, even though the depression itself testifies to the existence of an unconscious phantasy of having already devoured the ambivalently regarded object. A second example is the phantasy of containing the container of the self, as in the instance of maintaining a sense of contact with the 'containing' analyst during separations by imagining that one has incorporated the analyst; in this instance, Euclidean space is inadequate to the job of mapping out the domain of unconscious phantasy. A third example is the adult male phantasy of being both a boy and a girl and also both the child and the parent of his parents.

It is probably never fully warranted to claim with certainty that one understands and can designate exactly the sequence or hierarchy of phantasies pertaining to incorporation. Technically, it seems, there is much to be gained by the analyst's tolerating the contradictoriness of many unconscious phantasies and conveying that tolerance to the analysand. The alternative of making too much order among unconscious phantasies is most likely to support intellectualisation and the analysand's idealisation of the analyst as omniscient or omnipotent. Tolerance of contradiction need not entail launching chaotic barrages of interpretation, or substituting what is merely thinkable as a possibility for what is strongly implied in the ongoing analytic dialogue or otherwise shown in the interaction.

Do we require the concept of *partial* incorporation, as Abraham seemed to think? I believe so. Although our view of unconscious phantasy is that it is predisposed toward all-or-none, black-or-white, and *pars pro toto* thinking, and although, in self-contradiction, unconscious phantasy may include partial and total incorporation at the same time, there does seem to be value in reserving some interpretations for what is primarily partial; for example, incorporation of only a penis, a breast, a damaged leg, or blind eyes. Again, making false choices and acting on too great a need for order may lead the analyst astray or limit the effectiveness of his or her analytic work. An example of usefully mixing the partial and the total would be the following: a female analysand unconsciously phantasises during holidays that, because the analyst does not think of her, she no longer exists, so that in her subjective experience and actions she feels deadened for the duration; she may be said to have incorporated the analyst as an empty container, which in one respect is totalistic but in another respect only partial in that it allows the analyst to be away and to have a mind filled with other things and people. There is no single correct way to take up this partial/total phantasy; more than one approach to it may be necessary.

Similarly, the placement of the phantasised figure need not be fixed or limited to one spot. A figure may be inside and outside simultaneously, as in the melancholic's simultaneously representing the object as already incorporated and as being kept outside. Also, depending on (or manifesting) changes in attitude, the locale of the figure may shift rapidly from inside to outside and back again. For example, a dreaded incorporation may seem to have taken place when the analyst's figure is unexpectedly experienced as being within, this then quickly followed by that figure's expulsion or reprojection and its characterisation as repugnant. In the analysis of transference, the locale of the analyst cannot be taken for granted; in the same way, owing to projective identification, the locale of the self or some aspect of it, such as understanding or feeling, may not remain effectively and consistently 'within'.

Case Example 1

Mr A, a young man, son of a highly demanding, critical, competitive father, manifested extensive disruption of cognitive functions. He could not perceive accurately, remember with certainty, or communicate with any clarity what he had encountered in his studies, social relationships, or activities. Approximate locutions such as 'something like that' and 'in a way' filled his analytic communications. He misremembered numbers, and he mispronounced words and names. Almost invariably he recalled the analyst's comments in a distorted way. It seemed that 'blocked incorporation' was a useful designation of the phantastic foundation of many of these phenomena. Because it was important to the analysand not to become like his father, blocking any incorporation of, and subsequent introjective identification with, father seemed to have a very high priority. In this case, one primary motive seemed to be to enact a castrated role in relation to his father and, in the analysis, to his analyst. This castrated role lived out the negative identity unconsciously being deposited in him by the father's projective identifications.

Enacting this role was also to engage in a form of warfare with the father, experienced in this connection as a demander of achievement. Additionally, the analysand's cognitive impairment seemed to blind him to evident limitations in the father's actual professional and social achievements; thereby, he was protecting the 'fragile father' whose fragility was supposed to be entirely lodged in him. This fragility included 'feminine' or 'castrated' aspects of the father's self now being enacted by the patient in his characteristic mode of function. He played all of this out in his transference and tried to stimulate countertransference of a 'paternal' type.

I have presented only enough of this patient's total emotional situation to show that incorporation of the father's aggressiveness and weakness both had and had not taken place, and that this contradictory state of affairs in the analysand's self was in the service of his seeking some equilibrium in his internal world. It is implied that a certain amount of introjective identification had developed in the wake of those incorporations that did take place.

Case Example 2

This young man had fought his way out of a rigidly Marxist upbringing. He had felt 'brainwashed' by that upbringing, indicating by his use of the term 'brainwashed' the interiority of the fanatical parental pressures. Also, he felt under constant surveillance and criticism, in which respect he was subject to the experience of presences in the form of eyes upon him and voices at him. For a time during his adolescence, he had been a firm believer in his parents' creed; later he had become 'disillusioned' and had 'broken away from them'.

In the course of analysing his struggle against feelings in the transference, it emerged that he was trying to believe that, in effect, he had purged himself (his internal world) of a variety of controlling and persecutory part-and whole-figures. Consequently, he believed that if he let the analyst become important to him and certainly if he let himself feel the analyst's presence within him, it would culminate in a repetition of brainwashing and willing bondage. This outcome he was determined to prevent. This incorporation had to be blocked. It did, therefore, occasion brief panic whenever he noted, as time went on and rapport grew, a sense of the analyst's presence with him or in him. He would then stabilise himself by launching into scathing critiques of the idealism of psychoanalysis, the bourgeois values of psychoanalysts, and the personal faults of his analyst. Beyond expulsion, a wall of disgust had to be erected, in order, he hoped, to block any further ingestion. Also, a wall of negative countertransference, if possible.

Case Example 3

Ms C's mother had been severely depressed and hospitalised on more than one occasion, some of them early in the analysand's life. In the analysis, this young woman gave signs of having attempted desperately to repress her incorporation of her mother. Blocking incorporation in general seemed to have become a general strategy of life. Her mother had seemed to view the world around her and all the figures in it, including the analysand, with distaste. This distaste was covered with a shallow show of benevolence.

The young woman carried over this distaste, looking at the world through her mother's (incorporated) eyes in what might be regarded as a partial identification. But she also felt that she had to be wary of engaging in incorporation in relation not only to her mother but to all other 'maternal' figures, including the analyst, for all were regarded as forces of noxious (depressive) influences. Thus, her attack on incorporation was two-pronged and powerful. Her strategy in the analysis was this: to hold the analyst at bay by affectlessness. This affectlessness would also serve, she hoped, to protect the analyst from rude surprises, such as unsettling shows of feeling or independence; in part, that same concerned mode of function had been developed to protect the fragile mother. Thus, the analyst as depressive mother was both being held at bay and being protected, and additionally was being regarded as repugnant just as the analysand had been by her mother. Like her mother, she was superficially compliant, but her compliance was thin even though firmly in place.

More so than in the cases of Mr A and Mr B, this analysand fought against incorporation in the transference with great success. Almost entirely, she made use of the analyst only from a great psychic distance; she improved her lot to some extent and then stood pat until the analysis was ended.

I believe that for this analysand the greatest fear of all was the uncovering of the already incorporated, depressively mad mother. While the character trait of distaste could be analysed with some effect, approaches to the other major issues usually led to increased freezing of feeling, some suspiciousness, and regression to other symptomatic positions that, over time, had been relieved. They had been relieved by the combination of analytic work closer to the surface and the achievement of some differentiation of the analyst from the malignant mother and some more realistic incorporation of him, a combination that allowed her to derive a limited amount of support from the analytic relationship.

To summarise: I organised my presentation around the clinically valuable concept of blocked incorporation. Interpreting unconscious phantasies of incorporation, achieved or blocked, is a subtle, often seemingly contradictory enterprise. The conception of unconscious phantasy as fluid, non-Euclidean, illogical, fragmented, and concretistic, which should be an essential part of every analyst's equipment, is never more needed than in working out the vicissitudes of anti-incorporative strategies. These strategies play major roles in structuring and limiting transference and the analysand's designs on the countertransference. Several brief case examples were adduced to illustrate these complexities.

Good learning from others cannot do without substantial contributions of one's own, but these contributions cannot come to much without those core ideas and attitudes one incorporates from good teachers and good models, Hanna Segal being an outstanding example of both virtues.

References

Abraham, K. (1916) 'The First Pregenital Stage of the Libido', in *Selected Papers on Psychoanalysis*, New York: Basic Books, (1954), pp. 248-79.

—— (1921) 'Contributions to the Theory of the Anal Character', in *Selected Papers of Karl Abraham*, New York: Basic Books, (1953), pp. 337-92.

Freud, S. (1905) 'Three Essays on the Theory of Sexuality', *S.E.*, 7: 123-243, London: Hogarth Press, (1953).

—— (1917) 'Mourning and Melancholia', *S.E.*, 14: 237-58, London: Hogarth Press, (1957).

Schafer, R. (1968) *Aspects of Internalisation*, New York: International Universities Press.

—— (1972) 'Internalisation: process or fantasy?', *The Psychoanalytic Study of the Child*, 51: 265-8.

8

Enclaves and Excursions

Edna O'Shaugnessy

I wish to call attention to two hazards for the analyst intrinsic to the conduct of psychoanalysis. I shall name these 'enclaves' and 'excursions'. In the course of clinical work an analyst may be at risk of so responding to his patient that he forms an enclave, or takes an excursion out of analysis, and thereby deforms the psychoanalytic situation so that the therapeutic process is interfered with or even halted.

Enclaves

I shall first illustrate what I mean by an 'enclave' by describing the case of Miss A. An attractive woman in her thirties, Miss A wanted an analysis because, though successful in her career, her relationships with men were impermanent and her biological time was running out. At the start of the analysis, she and I seemed well attuned. An intricate exchange took place between us about her feelings and thoughts about herself, the new analysis and her analyst. These explorations were, in their way, valid, though I was aware after a while of the lack of unconscious depth in Miss A's communications, and how very personal, even intimate, her generally appreciative relationship to me was, and that while she expressed also some aggression, it had no real punch – though my sense of Miss A was of someone with powerful feelings.

I found I did not know what Miss A's unconscious phantasies were, or who or what I was as a transference object, or what connections there were between the analysis and her past history. I made some tentative attempts to speak of myself as a transference figure, e.g. I referred to myself as a 'mother-analyst' and I also tried to link events of the analysis with Miss A's history, by saying, e.g. that she felt now as she had when her brother was born. These interpretive attempts did not convince my patient and they led to no development. I stopped them as inauthentic

147

and was driven back to interpreting in the denuded 'you-me, me-you' way.

Reflecting on this analytic situation, I saw that I had mistaken, just as Miss A herself does, over-closeness for closeness, and mistaken, too, a restrictive and restricting part-object relationship for full contact between whole persons. My dissatisfaction with the 'you-me' interpretations that I had been making was now clearer. These interpretations were not part of a full interpretation, which in principle could eventually be completed, and involve internal objects, the interplay between unconscious phantasy and reality, and the reliving of the past. These interpretations were intrinsically denuded of such connections. They were part of the opening interaction between Miss A and myself, which both constituted and facilitated the emergence of Miss A's characteristic relations to her objects.

However, had I continued to interpret in the same way, I would be in danger of making what I am proposing to call an 'enclave' with Miss A. More aware, instead of bypassing these problems with interpretations of myself as the mother-analyst or making at this point inevitably artificial parallels with my patient's history, I stayed with the uncomfortable fact that I could not see who I was in the transference, that there were no links available to Miss A's history, and that her and my outside life seemed not to exist. I tried to explore and analyse Miss A's limited and over-close relationship to me, and my own denuded functioning with her – an exploration which Miss A both resisted and wanted.

I think some degree of acting out by the analyst inevitably occurs as a relationship like Miss A's with her objects emerges in the analysis. Once the analyst is able to see it for what it is, however, the analyst's shift in internal perspective brings about a corresponding shift in the style and content of his interpretations, which helps to change the analytic situation from emergence of the patient's problems with unwitting enactment by the analyst, to emergence with potential for containment and transformation by the analyst.

With more awareness, I could help Miss A to see the true nature of her relationship to me. When there were relevant dynamic indications in her material, I spoke about her over-gentleness and over-closeness, her exclusion of other life, hers and mine, present and past, her control and impoverishment of me, and anxieties about herself and myself which seemed to lie behind her need for so limited and limiting a contact, which, as we now saw, stopped the analyst from disturbing Miss A and Miss A from disturbing the analyst. As time went on, Miss A found she was not entirely free of disturbance: she felt more anxious in sessions, and she was able to feel and express real disappointment and resentment.

Important unconscious phantasies emerged. She had

> a dream of homosexual seclusion, in which two figures, like a pair of erotised instruments, played and touched each other, so that there was no discord between them.

Miss A's over-close, secluded relationship with me was thus revealed as a homosexual refuge, an erotised intimacy between similar, highly attuned instruments. Miss A was alarmed at the homosexuality, but very relieved by the interpretation of the mutual touching and playing in her dream, as the placation she felt was necessary between her and me for fear that, otherwise, we might become violent to each other.

For defensive and other purposes our patients need to make refuges of various sorts. We see at once that a delicate technique is called for from the analyst, a technique which both accepts a patient's need to make a refuge of the analytic situation, but, at the same time, analyses it. In this way the analyst averts the danger of so becoming what the patient requires that he deforms into an enclave what should be an analysis. Our patients feel, quite rightly, that the analysis of their refuge will change it, and bring exposure to what they fear they or their objects – in the analysis, the analyst – will not be able to bear.

As important as not enacting an enclave with a patient is not pushing and forcing a patient out of his refuge. Scrutiny of Miss A's dream tells us that within her refuge she has split off fears of seductive similarities between herself and her objects; the fact that she makes a refuge of symmetry and over-closeness tells us that she is even more afraid of differences and distance between herself and her objects. In sessions when acute anxiety threatened, Miss A worked to rebuild her refuge, subtly and powerfully controlling me to be over-close and to operate within its limits, and I had to struggle again with the difficult problem of how to interpret to minimise acting out with her.

At other times Miss A was ready to broaden her contact and to reach towards new areas. We know defensive formations change only with the strengthening of the ego, and that interpretations must not breach needed defences, but respect and acknowledge them. Nor, however, should interpretations lag behind what our patient's ego is ready for – notwithstanding the resistance we also know we must expect: to facilitate growth we must be timely with the new.

Interpretations made at the beginning of Miss A's analysis had two functions. They allowed for the emergence of her need for a refuge of homosexual seclusion, and the interpretations themselves gave her the restricted and undisturbing contact she required. However, had I remained unaware that Miss A was all the time drawing me into making denuded, undisturbing interpretations and had I continued interpreting in the same way, I would have gone on to provide Miss A, not with an analysis, but with an enclave.

According to Bion (1963), a psychoanalytic interpretation should have extension in the domains of sense, myth and passion. Miss A had needed me to make interpretations denuded of myth and passion, because of her fears of knowing her personal myths (her unconscious phantasies and world of inner objects), and of knowing her passions (her instincts and feelings). By keeping us over-close, denying our differences, obliterating the analyst's life beyond sessions and excluding also her own current life from her sessions (the counterpart in the analysis of how, in life, she dared not marry and have children) out of fear – all of which we gradually discovered – of the enviously depriving passions of her objects, Miss A constructed a denuded situation.

As a transference figure, I was an analyst who was no analyst, the denuded successor of a mother Miss A saw as no mother, and a father she saw as no father. She did not expect me to be willing to accept or to be able to stand her impulses, or to be capable of understanding her. Once I was more sensitive to the nature of the relationship Miss A really had made with me, I could try to analyse these unconscious presumptions and anxieties.

In sum: Miss A began her analysis by transferring into the analytic situation her restricted object relations. She communicated with words and non-verbal projections to help me to understand her and to control me to be the analyst with whom it would be possible for her to function. In accepting my transference role, I, to an extent, became the too well-attuned, over-close and denuded object she needed as a refuge from the fuller and freer object relations she unconsciously feared.

For me there was in this situation an inherent danger of being drawn too much into my patient's world and, in this way, letting the analysis actually become the symbolic equivalent of mildly erotised, symmetrical homosexual relations. I would then have made an enclave (as I propose to call it) of circumscribed contact, in which, though we continue trying to know about our interaction, our efforts stay within the restricted limits prescribed by the refuge. Until this situation is changed by the analysis of it, little therapeutic progress will be made.

8. Enclaves and Excursions

Excursions

An enclave deforms an essential feature of a psychoanalysis – its openness to possibilities of disturbance and the knowing of new areas. An excursion is different – not to do with limiting what is faced and known, but with totally evading emotional contact because of a terror of knowing.[1] Take a simple example of a threatened excursion familiar to every analyst: on the threshold of new emotional events, a patient quickly says: 'You mean, I can't stand separateness and dependence'. Though it is true he has problems with separateness and dependence, we all know how important it is not to discuss these at such a moment – that is, not to go on an excursion, but, instead, to draw the patient's attention to how, out of fear of the new, unknown emotional situation, he is trying to move himself and his analyst away to old and familiar ground.

Some patients besiege the analyst to go on excursions with them. I shall describe Mrs B who made repeated desperate attempts to move away from the incoherent experience of her sessions and take us instead on an excursion of pseudo-sense. A previous therapy had ended with Mrs B actually taking her therapist away on holiday with her. With me, there was a first six months of cautious enquiry, and then she let out into the analysis confused, ill, hyper-mobile areas of herself and her objects. These, for a long period, dominated the transference situation.

The pattern of her sessions was roughly as follows. In relation to some event in her life or the analysis, Mrs B would mention the names of a few persons and places of residence, and her feelings of anxiety or depression, moving rapidly from one item to the next. She seemed to some degree absent from what she was talking about. The identity of the people and places mentioned shifted in even a few sentences, so that her session was quickly cluttered and confusing. Though the same names and places tended to occur in session after session, it was nearly impossible for me to know who, in Mrs B's world, was who, what was internal or external, phantasy or reality.

I spoke to her about her anxious shifting, her need to communicate the flux and mental confusion she was suffering; her need, also, to keep out of contact with what she was talking about. Often after these initial interpretations I did not know what further to say, and I would fall silent and wait. Mrs B then became extremely anxious and felt I was dismissing what she had said. Tension increased. She conveyed an urgency of demand for me to do something and I would review what she had told me and try to think, in relation to the atmosphere of that

151

day, where her emotional centre might lie. Was she preoccupied with one of the people she had mentioned? Was it the state of the analyst? Or her own mind? Or the coming weekend? Etc., etc.

With a feeling of relief, I would select and pursue some theme. This brought relief to my patient also, but usually only temporarily. Mostly Mrs B would soon be on the move, away from the theme I was interpreting. I was then uncertain whether her movements away were because I was wrong, or were her rejection of my being right, or were less specific and expressed her pervasive mistrust of me. We often ended with a sense of nothing accomplished. After such a session, moreover, anxieties reverberated in me: I felt guilty of appalling work, I feared I had addressed the wrong issues, I feared Mrs B would not return (at the same time I knew she was not about to break off treatment). Then I shifted to another view: surely the session had not been so disastrous, had not this bit or that been in touch? And so on. That is, post-session, just like my patient, I had anxious, shifting states of mind.

After some months, I saw that this pattern was repeating itself and that there was no movement in the analysis. Contact with Mrs B was minimal and the minimal moments were not sustained. Nor was Mrs B contained; I and the sessions were too small for the scale of all her psychic operations. Many of her projections arrived in me, not during, but after, her sessions, when I endured the same anxious flux that tormented her. In sum, there was little contact and I, as analyst, was effecting no modification.

I began to think that the terrible tension which mounted at a certain point in Mrs B's sessions and which had driven me to find a theme to talk about was really latent panic, in me and in her, that I was unable to modify her mental state. Instead of going on what were really excursions into pseudo-sense with some 'theme', I started to focus on my failure to give her relief or effect any change. Mrs B was openly grateful when I understood this, even though it increased her anxiety, because while she felt understood, she at the same time experienced me as thrusting at her 'the fact' that analysis was useless for her.

Next, she had two dreams, followed by an important concrete proposal for mutual acting out. Her dreams, unlike many of her previous dreams, were significant in not being themselves a flight from psychic reality, but, on the contrary, a movement towards trying to know what was happening between us. In the first dream,

Mrs B was in a city, trying to get into two churches, which were stuffed

full with things of all sorts. In the dream, she was also always in the wrong
place at the wrong time.

Her dream expresses her predicament. She is trying to reach and get
into herself and me, represented by the two churches, but she is
obstructed because both of us are full of clutter, as indeed we truly were.
In the dream, Mrs B recognises how she is further frustrated by her own
flights and absences of mind – she feels she is never in the right place at
the right time in relation to herself or me. In her session Mrs B was well
in touch with the validity of her dream and its insights.

A few days later she began her session by speaking with perplexity
about her superior at work, after which she related a second insightful
dream.

> She was in her garden. A lorry arrived to deliver a huge load of glass
> cloches. In the dream she felt total incomprehension, because the cloche
> frames were weak and their glass was cracked. She could not understand
> why cracked, broken cloches were dumped on her, since she already had
> plenty of cloches like that herself.

This dream portrays more images of herself and her objects. She sees
her objects as being uncohesive (like a heap of cloches), and impervious
(glassy), mad (cracked), and with feeble containment (the weak frames).
They are like herself in these ways, and it is incomprehensible to her
that they should unload on to her their psychic states, huge and identical
to her own.

I first related Mrs B's dream to the superior at work she had
mentioned at the start, about whom she felt such perplexity, and then
I connected it to her view of myself and what I do to her when I talk to
her. At first she was glad I was not glassed off about the meaning of her
dream and thankful that I understood her incomprehension about the
relations between heedless people, especially her panic about being
projected into. Later a different idea took her over: I was dumping my
cracked ideas of human relations on her. She lost her feeling of being
understood and on succeeding days she was increasingly persecuted and
anxious.

An intense session then took place during unusually lovely summer
weather. Half-way through, with a mixture of uncertainty and despair
in her voice, Mrs B said: 'What would you do if I stretched my hand
backwards and touched you? If I said: "Come! Let's go and stand on
the bridge and watch the trains go by. Let's get out of here into the
sunshine".' Mrs B was in earnest. She was testing whether I would or

would not accept her invitation to quit analysis. The session was intense as I talked about her fears that I was either in despair, or cracked and corrupt, and might really choose to enjoy the weather with her rather than work. I interpreted that her proposal expressed her despair, too, and, also her hope that we might not move out of analysis into the sunshine, but stay to try to know the meaning of her proposal.

Indeed, Mrs B's proposal was an aid to understanding, both in the session itself and also because I saw how invitations 'to go out into the sunshine' had occurred in subtler forms before, during those silences when tension rose and I felt an enormous pressure to do something with what Mrs B had told me. I realised even more clearly that when I found myself looking for an emotional centre in the content of Mrs B's material and chose a theme to talk about, though this relieved me and also gave Mrs B a little (usually temporary) relief, this was an excursion out of analysis into pseudo-normality away from the truth that she had no emotional centre, that her ego was in fragments, that she urgently needed its repair and feared I was unable to do it.

Now, at such times, I spoke about the atmosphere of mutual anxiety that we had come again to what felt like an impasse. I spoke about her fear that she and I were in the same uncohesive and cluttered state, and I addressed her panic that instead of healing her mind, I might make her worse by offloading my own state into her. I tried, of course, to analyse each of these areas in terms of the variable details of a given day.

Over a long period, Mrs B's level of anxiety dropped substantially; she ceased to be in continual flight from herself and her objects, nor was her mind in a state of perpetual confused flux; except for rare returns in special circumstances, post-session reverberations ceased in myself. Every analyst knows how stressful analysis is for such a patient, and how, though better, the patient continues to face formidable difficulties, as does, in a different way, the analyst.

Conclusion

To review the case of Mrs B: Mrs B was a patient whose chief defence – hyper-mobility to avoid contact – increased her distressed state of flux and confusion. As psychic items were passed back and forth between us without being modified, she pressured me to move away from these incoherent object relations and make, instead, interpretations of pseudo-sense. In this way, Mrs B externalised into the analysis her mental world where there existed an underlying psychotic matrix that she and her objects were in terror of facing and kept avoiding. Once I realised that my resolution of crucial tensions between us by looking for normal themes in the content of her material was really an evasion of her panic that I was no help to her, and began to talk to Mrs B about this, a very important shift occurred which enabled her underlying psychotic condition to emerge in its full complexity. The real level of Mrs B's problems could then begin to be addressed.

It is obvious that had I continued, even in far less gross modes than 'going out into the sunshine', to succumb to her chronic pressure to go on joint flights, there could have been little advance in Mrs B's analysis. Her deep pathology would have been bypassed, not only by her, which was her right, but by me, which would have been my wrong. I would then have deformed an analysis into a series of excursions. Mrs B, you will recall, actually took a previous therapist away on holiday with her – a fact which shows the formidable force she exerts and which the analyst has to withstand.

Going on excursions with patients, or forming an enclave with them, are among the hazards intrinsic to the therapeutic endeavour. James Strachey, in his classic paper 'The nature of the therapeutic action of psychoanalysis' (1934), called attention to how 'the analytic situation is all the time threatening to degenerate into a "real" situation'. He continued:

> But this actually means the opposite of what it appears to. It means that the patient is all the time on the brink of turning the real, external object (the analyst) into the archaic one; that is to say, he is on the brink of projecting his primitive introjected images onto him. In so far as the patient actually does this ... (the) analyst then ceases to possess the peculiar advantages derived from the analytic situation (p. 284).

Strachey is referring to the very phenomenon which is the subject of this paper: the inbuilt risk of degeneration in a psychoanalytic situation. Strachey's notion of the patient 'trying to turn the analyst into an archaic object' is nowadays one aspect of accepted interactional clinical thinking, as over the years the psychoanalytic view of patient and analyst shifted away from exploring in isolation either the patient or the analyst and towards exploring in depth their interaction. Langs in *The Therapeutic Interaction* (1976) has summarised and discussed the writings of many analysts from different schools who have contributed to this overall change, and, though it is conceptualised variously, analysts over a wide spectrum continue to explore patient-analyst interaction.

This contemporary context is the general background of the present paper. Very relevant, for instance, is Schafer's (1959) important concept of generative empathy, and Ezriel's (1980) account of the tension the patient feels with the analyst between the required relationship and the avoided one. My more specific understanding of the way the patient interacts with the analyst is based on the concept of projective identification, as extended by Bion (1957, 1959) to encompass the defences and impulses described by Melanie Klein (1952) and, also, his own discovery of projective identification as the earliest mode of communication. Spillius (1988) has a valuable discussion of projective identification in her introduction to the topic in *Melanie Klein Today*, while clinical studies of the patient's projective identifications into the analyst – both to communicate and to control him to act out a particular role – have been done most notably by Joseph (1989).

In my experience, because of the communicative and controlling functions of the patients' projective identifications, some acting out by the analyst inevitably occurs. Sandler (1976), with a different theory, has also pointed out how enactment by the analyst occurs as part of emergence in the transference situation of the patient's unconscious primary object relations. Carpy (1989) draws attention, with a different emphasis, to the importance for the patient of the analyst's partial acting out.

If the analysis is not to degenerate, it is vital that such partial acting out by the analyst is recognised, contained and analysed. These contentions disagree both with the view that if only the analyst were more quickly more aware he could entirely avoid acting out with his patient, and also with the view that acting out beyond the very limited and partial amount necessary for emergence, and to accommodate to what the patient can bear, can be beneficial. My two cases, plus some conceptual considerations, are offered as evidence of the existence of an inbuilt risk, with certain patients, of the analyst deforming the analysis into some type of enclave or excursion which will hinder or halt therapeutic progress, such risks being all the more insidious because some limited, partial acting out with the patient can play a valuable part in revealing what the transference relationship is. As Segal (1987) remarks: 'The same factors which are the crux of a potentially therapeutic situation also have a potential for an anti-therapeutic one'.

In addition to work during sessions, an analyst needs time to reflect on the overall interaction between himself and his patient, to consider the question of change and repetition, to think about his feelings for and his ways of behaving with and speaking to his patient. Whether he and his patient are keeping out disturbances, and whether they tend to move away from, rather than towards, 'trying to know'. Such reflection can help the analyst to be more aware of the overall transference situation and to work with less acting out and more insight.

Miss A and Mrs B each illustrate one type of enclave and excursion. With Miss A, I was at risk of enacting the analytic equivalent of a homosexual enclave. With other patients, there might, for example, be the risk of turning the analysis into an enclave of mutual idealisation, or libidinised despair, or concealed psychotic phantasy. There are many sorts of enclaves and excursions and patients are not necessarily exclusively of one type or the other.

For excursions, I chose the case of Mrs B as an extreme and therefore vivid illustration. With her I was always at risk of evading her severe difficulties by moving off into pseudo-coherence and normality. With a less ill patient the risk of excursions occurs not continually but at times of special anxiety, when the patient may try to induce the analyst to foreclose with a pat interpretation, or give practical guidance or have an intellectual discussion; or the patient may unconsciously manoeuvre the analyst into moralising, disciplining or reassuring him, or into speculating about (as opposed to true analytic reconstruction of) his past. All of these exemplify excursions away from some point of analytic urgency in the session.

Before concluding I wish to discuss one seemingly interminable dispute: the debate about transference versus extra-transference interpretations. Naturally, but I think mistakenly, anxiety about analysis being deformed into an enclave has fastened exclusively onto the use of transference interpretations; similarly, anxiety about analysis degenerating into a series of excursions has fastened exclusively onto the use of extra-transference interpretations. The thesis of this paper is that both hazards are intrinsic to the conduct of an analysis with patients like Miss A and Mrs B, irrespective of any particular analytic approach.

Many authors – for example recently Stewart (1990), but more extensively Blum (1983) – have written of their concern that interpreting solely in the transference turns an analysis into an over-close enclave. Their presumption is that by focusing on what has sometimes been called the 'here and now', the analyst degenerates into a type of 'you-me, me-you' interpreting, which retreats from its proper analytic function and neglects events, even urgent events, in the patient's current life, and also ignores the patient's history, so that analysis becomes the patient's only life – really a retreat from life.

However, as illustrated by the case of Miss A, an over-close refuge between patient and analyst occurred, not because of my particular technique, but because it was the necessary externalisation in the

157

transference of her characteristic relations with her objects. Had a different approach been used – say, of encouraging Miss A to recall and to recount childhood memories – she would unconsciously have attuned herself to *that* analyst, and controlled that analyst to interpret her history in a way that did not disturb her. She would again have established a refuge of restricted contact, homosexual in nature, this time in relation to her past.

This is not to say there could not be a poor interpretive technique which fosters what Blum calls 'a *folie-à-deux*' and what I call 'an enclave'. Indeed, one of my chief points is exactly that. If the analyst remains unaware of the nature of the archaic relationship his patient draws him into, and continues to enact it and not analyse it, there will, indeed, be a *folie-à-deux*. As remarked above, in a parallel way, the fear of going on excursions has historically attached itself exclusively to the technique of extra-transference interpretations, whereas, in fact, this hazard is intrinsic to all analytic situations in which a patient is in terror of knowing and desperate to take flight from contact.

Whatever our different psychoanalytic techniques, we share a concern not to deform an analysis into an enclave or a series of excursions. In practice it is often on these grounds that we reject one way of interpreting and choose another. When we discuss different ways of talking to our patients, I think it more useful, rather than asking whether an interpretation is a transference or extra-transference interpretation, to explore the interaction between patient and analyst, so as to see the nature of their contact. We should ask, importantly, whether the analyst's technique wards off rather than permits the entry of what is new and disturbing, and whether the type of movement being made by patient and analyst is towards or away from 'trying to know'. This, I think, is more in keeping with our contemporary interactional perspective.

A last word. Enclaves and excursions differ in a fundamental way. A patient who makes an enclave feels there is some way he can relate to an object – provided he finds an already suitable object or reshapes an object to fit what he requires to keep out aspects which threaten him with too much anxiety. Such patients find some way of making contact with their analyst. The patient who goes on excursions is different. He believes no manageable contact is possible with his object and the level of his anxiety is horrendous. Contact must be evaded, a new situation constructed, which characteristically in its turn becomes untenable. These patients are hyperactive, their talk proliferates, as, typically, do their dream images.

8. Enclaves and Excursions

Mrs B is an example of a patient threatened with anxiety so acute she is all the time near to panic. Hers is a psychotic matrix, i.e. a matrix of object relations in which she believes no amelioration is possible. In analysis she is impelled to perpetual flights from herself and her analyst. Even in its less severe manifestations, a patient's impulse to pull the analyst on a joint flight away from attempts 'to try to know' signals terror about the state of the self, or the analyst, or both, which means that potential contact is very dangerous indeed. Copyright © Institute of Psycho-Analysis.

Notes

1. Balint (1959) distinguished two defensive character types, the ochnophil who clings to his objects, and the philobat who avoids them. Although our distinctions are not quite congruent, Balint's ochnophil is similar to the patient with whom the analyst risks making an enclave, and his philobat is like the patient with whom there is a risk of turning the analysis into a series of excursions.

References

Balint, M. (1959) *Thrills and Regressions*. London: Hogarth.

Bion, W. (1957) 'Differentiation of the psychotic from the non-psychotic personalities', *International Journal of Psychoanalysis*, 38: 266-75. Also in *Second Thoughts*. London: Heinemann, (1967); repr. London: Karnac Books, (1984).

—— (1959) 'Attacks on linking', *International Journal of Psychoanalysis*, 40: 308-15. Repr. in *Second Thoughts*, London: Heinemann, (1967).

—— (1963) *Elements of Psycho-Analysis*, London: Heinemann. Repr. in the Maresfield Library (1984).

Blum, H.P. (1983) 'The position and value of extra-transference interpretations', *Journal of the American Psychoanalytic Association*, 31: 587-617.

Carpy, D.V. (1989) 'Tolerating the countertransference: a mutative process', *International Journal of Psychoanalysis*, 70: 287-93.

Ezriel, J. (1980) *A Psychoanalytic Approach to Group Treatment in Psycho-Analytic Group Dynamics*, New York: International University Press.

Joseph, B. (1989) *Psychic Equilibrium and Psychic Change*, London: Routledge.

Klein, M. (1952) 'Notes on Some Schizoid Mechanisms', in *Developments in Psycho-Analysis*, (ed.) J. Riviere, London: Hogarth.

Langs, R. (1976) *The Therapeutic Interaction*, Vols 1, 2, New York: Jason Aronson.

Sandler, J. (1976) 'Countertransference and role responsiveness', *International Journal of Psycho-Analysis*, 57: 43-8.

Schafer, R. (1959) 'Generative empathy in the treatment situation', *Psycho-analytical Quarterly*, 28: 342-73.

Segal, H. (1987) *What is therapeutic and counter-therapeutic in psychoanalysis?*, (unpublished).

Spillius, E. (1988) *Melanie Klein Today*, vol. 1, London: Routledge.

Stewart, H. (1990) 'Interpretation and other agents for psychic change', *International Review of Psychoanalysis*, 17: 61-70.

Strachey, J. (1934) 'The Nature of the therapeutic action of psycho-analysis', *International Journal of Psycho-Analysis*, 15: 127-59. Repr., 50: 275-92.

'Where There Is No Vision'

From Sexualisation to Sexuality

Betty Joseph

Throughout her writing career Hanna Segal has always been particularly interested in freedom of thought and its relation to creativity, and the influence of her work can be seen on this paper. This contribution is essentially concerned with creativity – mental vision – based on the freedom to think and imagine, and its connection with mature sexuality as opposed to sexualisation.

Freud (1910) describes how sexualisation, erotisation of parts of the body prevents those parts from functioning properly, taking as his example that of vision. I want also to talk about vision, but mental vision, using the verse from Proverbs, 'Where there is no vision the people perish'. I shall connect this lack of vision and the resultant destruction of generations with the destruction of creativity. I want to discuss how sexualisation, which in the analytic situation means enactment, is in fact the antithesis of thinking, it is used by patients to avoid thought which they both hate and fear. I hope to show how sexualisation is employed as a defence against real relating, which implies separateness from the object, and thus against real sexuality. Without this sense of separateness and relating there can be no imaginative thought and no vision.

If we start from the core of our work, that is in the transference, we see erotisation operating to very different degrees. Some of the grossest examples Freud quoted in 1913, in his paper on 'Transference Love' describing how the patient erotises the transference, and is clearly aiming to seduce the analyst away from doing his job, to undermine the proper analytic relationship between patient and analyst and thus prevent creative work being done. The patient describes this as love, but the analyst soon recognises that it is deeply destructive.

We of course see other aspects of erotisation of the transference, in the whole range of the perversions, some obvious and gross, others more hidden and insidious and these in varying degrees will be acted out in the transference. I think it would be true to say that perversion is ubiquitous, it is not the prerogative of seriously ill borderline patients but will be found in the vast majority, if not all, of our seriously ill and many of our not so seriously ill patients.

I want now to give an example of a perverse element in the analysis of a not so seriously disturbed young woman, L, whose analysis terminated a few years ago when she left, possibly a bit prematurely, to take up work abroad. She had married when still a student, but very soon after the young couple divorced. L starts the session speaking self-consciously, indicating that I shall not approve of what she is thinking about. She has seen an excellent dress that she likes very much, but it is very expensive, she really needs one, has not bought any clothes for ages etc. (At this point I cannot help thinking to myself how she appears almost daily in something different, so must have quite an extensive wardrobe.) She continues haltingly and I can feel myself almost on the point of saying something to the effect of her knowing how much she has, and how she has been stressing her need to be very careful financially.

Then I realise that this is just what she has been waiting for, almost expecting. I point out to L that she seems to be telling me about the dress as if expecting me to take a moralising approach, however much it may be couched in interpretative language. Then she can feel hurt and I shall be experienced as harsh and punitive. L continues, almost pleadingly to point out that, although it is expensive, (no sum is mentioned) it would be a very good buy, would last a long time, could be worn over years, and she reminds me of an expensive coat she bought a few years ago and is still wearing constantly. I point out to her that she is talking as if I had not made any interpretation, but as if I had actually been accusing her in a hostile way. At this point she starts to listen and can then see how she has set up the situation to get herself hurt, and has reacted as if I had really hurt and accused her. She almost shuddered at what she had anticipated would be my cruel condemnation.

From this it can be seen that she has in a minor way built up a sadomasochistic relation between the two of us, in her mind; sexualised this conversation, and then the thought, should she buy the dress, could not be used for thinking. Moreover one can see here that the relationship with me that is being built up, is not one of a relationship with a woman who might be expected to understand and sympathise with a younger woman's interest in clothes, whether or not she could afford them – but one of a woman who is old and envious of her youth and attractiveness, a person who will criticise her, verbally beat her, and thus actually gratify her masochism.

When she is caught up in this masochism she does not have to feel any concern about the actual thing she is discussing, or any guilt about what she is trying to stir up in the analytic situation. When her thinking becomes erotised in this way she cannot think and see what is going on, and therefore there is no possibility of our relationship being thought-ful, creative, and in this sense sexual. Following my interpretations the patient ceased to feel what I was saying as an actual expression of my sadism, concretely expressed. The relationship changed and she could use insight: interpretations became interpretations. Thus symbolisation had taken the place of concrete thinking, (Segal, 1957) and L could start to think, even to sort out the actual dress problem realistically. When she was locked in the sadomasochistic relationship only perverse sexu-ality was possible. It was however a long time before the underlying emotions, the whole envious area, her suspicions about mine, or any understanding of her own could be explored. The sexualisation pro-tected her from having to open up this area of thinking. It also throws light on a particular problem in L's earlier relationships, especially in the early failed marriage which seems to have been of a very unhappy sadomasochistic type.

Going back to Freud – one can see in this example the way in which erotisation damages ego functioning, here – the capacity to think. When the patient projects parts of herself into her object and the object becomes confused with the self, there can be no distance between self and object, and no symbolisation and without it there can be no vision. If the attempt to draw the analyst into action, to beat her with words rather than to think, succeeds, then the whole situation becomes actu-alised and expressed concretely. Thus the analyst's capacity for vision too is stultified and no new ideas can issue.

Many patients carry this erotisation of thinking into their daily internal lives. L would use analytic insights in an *apparently* thoughtful way when she was alone, but what emerged when we started to look at this was that she continued to use bits of so-called understanding to attack herself with, acting the role of cruel analyst as well as pained patient, but not concerning herself with what might have been gained from her understanding or getting on with ordinary living. Although in this situation it looks as if the patient suffers from guilt, it is in fact an evasion of guilt. She is actually absorbed in excited gratification of her sadomasochism, which can lead to no development and no repairing. With this sexualisation of the relationship there can be no true marriage of two minds, with all the everyday difficulties this involves, no coming together of the analyst's and patient's minds, internally or externally unconscious result can only be barren, and the perverse rather than creative.

The psychopathology of certain patients I believe is based on the maintenance of that position – the maintaining of a barren state. It is an aspect of their whole personality organisation, and it is this that I want to go on to discuss taking as my example the case of Mr A, a man in whose analysis there appeared a particular and limited type of sexualisation, he himself being a somewhat asexual man. The sexualisation is ordinarily rather hidden but when it emerges it is clear that it is directly opposed to real sexuality and real relating. Mr A came into analysis in his early thirties because of a major disturbance in his sexual/emotional life. He had, he believed, for the first time in his life, 'fallen in love' with a girl colleague at work, he was deeply attracted by her. There was no actual physical sexual behaviour involved. She rejected him. He felt desperate, very guilty towards his wife and two young daughters and almost suicidal. I soon learned that his relationship with his wife was very thin emotionally and their sexuality very limited. When they did have intercourse it involved a kind of verbal sadomasochistic bantering, the wife taking the active teasing role. His social life was almost nil. His few contacts largely consisted of sad people, 'lame ducks', people in a worse position than he and his family, needing him for advice, company or help and eventually becoming irksome to him. He had phobias about travelling in trains and planes, food fads and was considerably over-weight, eating excessively – as we later discovered. He had very limited memories of his childhood or his parents. They never seemed to come through as individuals with personalities of their own, nor was there any sense of them as a couple.

In the analysis Mr A was obsessional and rigid but apparently compliant, co-operative and helpful, fitting in with times, holidays, fees etc. Before bringing any detailed material I want to summarise some of my thinking about this case as it emerged in the early years of the analysis and relates to our theme of sexualisation and sexuality. This is a man whose actual sexual life as well as his general relationships with people, is extremely limited. So also are his thinking, his interests and his hopes for the future. In terms of his personality organisation it soon became clear that he was a highly narcissistic and omnipotent man, controlled and controlling, self-satisfied and feeling a quiet superiority over others around him. He would bring material in a way which suggested that we already understood it, or that it referred to 'known' ideas so that the sessions could easily become repetitive or superficial. But he would also, as we saw with L, though perhaps in a more hidden way, bring material unconsciously aimed at getting a critical or hurtful interpretation – thus building a sadomasochistic type of relationship with me, in which I could be felt to be like his wife, verbally beating him.

This was similar to his use of his own thinking. He would very quickly be drawn into a critical or hostile inner activity, going over and over, in his mind, some fault that he had found or suspected in, say, a colleague; he would then, in his mind attack, the other person would reply, he would humiliate in return, the other respond with further attacks and he would go on and on with this in his head until he was completely caught up in it. (It is similar to the kind of masochistic 'chuntering' that we saw in L, when she would relentlessly use what had previously been insight to attack and criticise herself, getting excitedly caught up into the process.) With Mr A as with L this seems to be used to obviate areas of painful thinking or relating.

I have described how lacking in mature relationships and how isolated socially Mr A was, and in the analysis it could be seen that I, the analyst as a person, hardly existed. What I want to explore here is something of the nature of the personality organisation of this type of patient showing this combination of sexualisation and little mature sexuality or mature emotional relating.

I shall bring material from a recent period, that is some years into the treatment, when my patient was occasionally beginning briefly to face the very serious nature of his condition. But before I bring this I want to go back a year or two to mention the kind of insights that had been leading up to the recent material. I shall describe some fragments without at this point attempting to discuss the actual transference implications or my detailed interpretations.

At a period when an important theme had been Mr A's need to avoid any awareness of gaps or separateness, he came on a Monday telling that he had woken anxious, convinced that I was going to say that I was retiring. He added that the previous week he had noticed that I looked old and not well. (I had no awareness of being unwell) and he spoke of other people who were retiring, adding that he felt disrupted this week partly because he had little work to do, partly because of the change of times. (Very unusually I had asked him to come earlier on the Friday.) At this point he was doing something with his fingers and although he does it a great deal in the sessions, I suddenly became very much struck by it. He touches the tips of the fingers of one hand against the fingers of the other very softly and almost unceasingly. In this instance I think the notion of being away, disturbed and separate from me stirred up some need to be physically in contact. The movements were a quasi-masturbatory activity, touching and touching, and seemed to serve as a protection against or denial of the idea of separation and the awareness that I really am old and must at some point retire or die. This mastur-batory activity seems to have something in common with the mental chuntering, the going over and over things in his mind, that I referred to earlier.

The following session the problem of the awareness of separateness was taken a step further. He described how a friend, Alice, had phoned and told him that she was considering seeking more analysis, and wondered whether she should approach me, his analyst, about it. He really believed that I might see her and offer her a vacancy and he was deeply upset. But by the next day this rather normal reaction of jealousy and sense of being left out, had disappeared, he was no longer worried but started to talk in detail about Alice. He realised what a disturbed woman she was, but he described what a pull she exerted on him with the ideas of some kind of mutual sexuality which would be wonderfully free – but also the word 'perverse' came in somewhere. He added that he realised that he used to go to her for 'mental comfort' sometimes on the last day of the analytic term and further, a thing he had never told me before, he used to have an urge to buy pornographic literature then, but did not actually do so.

We could then establish his idea that Alice would invite him in, not just for 'mental comfort' but literally inside her body – the idea of mutual sex. It was clearly linked with his doing what he liked, with perversion and pornography. Yet, he added, this point about Alice is quite at odds with the reality – her flat is very stylish but also cold and sterile. It is not a couch on which one could do things together, it would crumple the cover. What I want to show here is the way in which for a moment Mr A could experience jealousy within a three person relation-ship (when he thought there was a risk of Alice coming to me), but then this, along with any sense of rejection or gap disappeared and he became absorbed in a phantasy of being physically, concretely, drawn into her body. But really getting inside a woman's body stirs up perverse phan-tasies of damage and abuse which inevitably leads to claustrophobic anxieties. Yet to be outside is to be cold and separated off and this must be avoided – the compromise solution is suggested by the quasi-masturbatory finger touching, skin to skin, neither separate nor completely inside. There is no real relating here either to me as a real person or to Alice herself, there is no real intercourse either mental or physical – no exchange.

This finger to finger relationship, neither separate nor really relating, one sees also in Mr A's rare friendships. He was, over years, strongly connected with a man whom he knew through their mutual work, a man Sam (who will come into the material I shall quote a bit later). Sam was at first rather admired but soon slipped into being almost a double, a twin of Mr A and then more and more he was felt as inferior and as dependent on Mr A. They used to phone each other constantly, probably daily, discussing and exchanging ideas on their projects. They never had any real social contacts, say with their families, nor were they close and intimate personally.

I want now to take this discussion of the nature of his personality and relationships a step further by bringing brief material from the period shortly before this last Christmas. The session on Monday had seemed helpful, I had been able to understand and show him more about the tendency in the session to withdraw from contact.

Mr A arrived on Tuesday saying that his stomach felt all knotted up; he was uneasy about his mother who had been ill, he could not trust her not to do things that would get her into difficulties, such as work round the house. Also she seemed to want their company more. I suggested that I was this person whom he felt wanted him to be in contact with me more, and who should be under his control not doing things, saying things that he had not planned and did not want to hear. He agreed that he did get annoyed and rejecting and that he had not expected what I had just interpreted. He went on to describe how it makes him feel worse, guilty, when I, the analyst, try to talk and he doesn't engage, he freezes. This referred to our discussion the previous day about his withdrawing. It is, he said, as if he is holding his life together, a thread, precarious, or he would break down. It is necessary to keep control but keeping smooth has become increasingly impossible, things break out so often. (This was a very unusual kind of remark, the notion of breakdown.) He went on to give examples from home, about unexpected things etc. which however kept the issue on a known, familiar level. Then he turned to describing a problem about a series of lectures he had been giving for a London college; he had been paid comparatively little, but had now been doing some costing and he planned to present the organising chairman with his proposition about payment. He was worried that they would think that he was asking too much. In previous years the chairman would get his pals to do odd lectures – this is not serious academic work, it needs a proper intellectual basis, adding that if he does the whole course he wants to be paid for it. He resents the situation as it is. This was said with some vehemence.

I tried to show Mr A his resentment that I have a serious intellectual contribution to make to our work and he feels the emotional cost of facing this is, and was yesterday, too great – this is a reference to the fear of breakdown, I think. I am not just a pal but different from him in my professional role. He agreed that there was resentment, it feels precarious, and he repeated his anxiety about the money. But he felt that it was worse than that and he described how his feelings were of 'desperation', and added that he felt afraid that I, the analyst, would take him over, penetrate his mind. When I agreed that I thought this was really a very great anxiety he replied 'when you speak there is panic, then I can do nothing but replay the last few words until they are neutered'. He went on to describe how he has to hold me back a bit or I will take over and then he will not know what is put into him, what is him and what is me. 'While I stand at the door of my mind I can have communication.' (This is not a way of speaking that either he or I have used before, and seemed absolutely genuine.) From this I felt we could understand more about his need to keep me at bay, talking on the level of intellectual explanations, with himself as the observer and gate keeper at what he calls the entrance of his mind, and then he can talk to and with me. But once he gives up gate-keeping the analyst might take over. He slowly added, 'I need you to help educate me, not invade'. Interestingly at this point I felt that things were beginning to go wrong and he was starting to push us into a kind of mutual defensive intellectualisation about something which moments before had been very real and very disturbing to him.

I then remained quiet, there was a pause and he added, 'I cannot talk to Sam, it will push me over the edge because I might tell him exactly what I think. He is aggrieved with me, I have not had any work for him although I've tried – he tries to make me feel I owe him something. If he presses me again I shall turn and snarl at him. For the last ten years or so I've kept him in business – his ingratitude – if I told him what I think our relationship couldn't continue'.

At the beginning of the session he did for a moment face that I have something to give that might enter his mind, and he resented it. But this resentment seems to be quite superficial compared with the acute underlying anxiety. In this material we can see a very important aspect of the patient's problems, namely his panic that when I speak something will get into his mind. I am then experienced as penetrating, invading, taking over until there will be confusion as to what comes from him, what from me? This panic must be defended against at all costs and so part of himself has to stand guard at the door of his own mind, neuter the words, freeze. This procedure enables him to hold his life together, thus evading, as he said, breakdown. The withdrawal, the blocking here is part of the whole defence against overwhelming 'desperation', panic, so there can be no real relating and exchange between us, no penetration, no receptivity, and therefore, as I would put it, no mental sexuality, only immobilisation and paralysis. Then there can be no vision or creativity, it is all blocked by the panic state.

Within this is, I think, the fear that I shall be driven into using force to penetrate his mind aggressively and really take over. With the blocking we both become neutered and symmetrical, a kind of bizarre homosexual couple, not a mutually creative couple. Towards the end of this material we can see other defences against the anxiety emerging, as he explains that he needs me to educate, i.e. explain, not invade, interpret. In the description of Sam he shows how he can get into my mind, take over my position, he then becomes the giver and I become like Sam, dependant on him for my work – understanding, and should thus be grateful to him. Then I become one of the lame ducks. Now we are on familiar ground. His defences are mobilised and the anxiety has for the moment disappeared but not been adequately dealt with.

However it reappeared in the following session as he started to describe how worried he was about the news of Michael Jackson and his alleged abuse of young people. But his greater worry concerned the treatment, the technique of the therapists treating him. Was Dr B involved? Dr B is a psychiatrist whom he, correctly, assumes I know. Something rotten is going on .... Now I could clearly show him the fear of myself as the therapist abusing, penetrating and manipulating him perversely, as he feels I do or will do, forcing my ideas into him. And I should add that, of course, it is more than possible that at times faced with his passivity and intellectualisations I may seem to push my interpretations at him. There is also the issue here of his wanting me to join in and be caught up in a kind of perverse excitement, interest or curiosity in the talk about Michael Jackson, so that we become a perverse analytically barren couple. Many of these elements seemed to come together in the following session when Mr A at the beginning of the session reported a dream,

> Mr A and his wife were at the theatre, far back, perhaps in the last row; there was a catwalk from the stage to the back. The play was of a Shakespearean type, it seemed dull and disappointing since it had had good reviews. There was a long dialogue between the main actors, a man and woman. The woman then flounced down along the catwalk, acting as though flirting with members of the audience as she passed. When she reached the level of the patient she climbed off and along the row,

ostensibly chatting with the audience. She seemed very taken with Mr A in a non-theatrical sense, she came over and kissed him. Something happened between them, they both became involved with each other.

In his associations Mr A said that it looked like a school hall, was supposed to be prestigious but it had an amateurish feeling. Yesterday a man at work, told about a bizarre happening. A woman psychiatrist from abroad had developed a one-sided attachment to a psychiatrist here, and was bombarding him with attention, had even turned up now in London! This was like the woman pestering him in the dream – except that in the dream he was involved too, it was real for him too. I thought that the whole dream must be connected with the previous sessions and queried whether he had not noticed this. After some pause he agreed that had gone through his mind. I had the feeling that the not mentioning had something provocative and teasing about it. He spoke about feeling irritated, he recognises the woman but cannot remember her name.

I made some tentative interpretations, and Mr A paused and went on apparently to a different topic. Yesterday he had an odd encounter with Mrs C (a very senior rather well known colleague). Because his own office is in a different building, he was, as he put it, camping in his secretary's office and working there. Mrs C came in and behaved towards him almost as if he could have been one of the secretaries. He felt such an outsider with all these people so busy and in their own offices, and he could have applied for a more central position earlier on.

To return to the dream, at the beginning Mr A has some awareness of being just in the audience, an observer at some distance. He and his wife are at the back of the hall watching the actors on the stage, in one sense himself and me; but it is also a couple in a serious dialogue with himself, he feels, left out. Again these are rather normal, sane feelings as we saw in the previous material when he briefly became jealous at the idea of my seeing Alice. These feelings have to be obliterated. The play has a good reputation but he found it boring and amateurish. (He knows that he was originally referred to me as a senior analyst with a good reputation.) He further degrades the situation and the main actress. She is sexualised, flounces down the catwalk, chats and is drawn to and kisses him, so both are involved, but he could not remember her name. He is no longer left out, any distance between him and the main characters has gone, he is no longer on the periphery, he is in the centre of his stage, the stage of his mind, with the main actress involved with him. The other man, the actor, representing my capacity to think, dialogue with myself, is cut out. It is interesting that the sexualisation

170

of the actress and his own involvement with her is felt by Mr A as real. I think that there is something that feels real to him in his relationship with me that I do not yet know sufficient about – is it that he does feel that I am particularly attracted to him in some way? He certainly has the idea that he is one of the few remaining patients that he believes I now have. I am clear that he is terrified of actually sexual involvement with an analyst, and that this is ordinarily split off from me as an external figure, by the reassurance that one of the reasons why he chose me was that given my age he would not be attracted to or get involved with me in the way he did with the girl colleague when he broke down, and the women like Alice.

We see both in the dream and in the material immediately following (namely about his being without an office and looked down on by Mrs C), how, the moment he is in touch with the feeling of being separate and relating to others, ideas about being an observer and alone become intolerable. They are dealt with by sexualising the experience, getting into the centre of the situation or becoming one of the couple, and the whole painful experience disappears. But of course, separateness, differentiation is an essential precursor to a coming together, to sexuality and all that this implies and this cannot be tolerated.

When I started to link the dream, especially the seductive element, to the previous session and his anxiety about the Michael Jackson case, and the therapists felt to be exploiting him in some perverse way, Mr A quickly said he had thought about that. He explained that he believed that one of the psychiatrists involved was a man whom he had consulted many years ago and who was involved professionally with many well know public figures, and this makes my patient feel on the periphery, lonely and left out. As I linked this with his fear of separateness and his need to get into the centre he moved slightly away and said that to him the important thing about being in the centre is being 'in the know'. But he added, now really thoughtfully, that for him being 'in the know' has something prurient about it. It was now the end of the session.

This point raises a further issue. When Mr A becomes aware that I have a separate mind, that my thoughts are not just ahead but different from his, and not centred on him, then he feels that he is concretely 'not in the know'. He tries to get into my mind, as in the dream he moved from being outside observer to becoming the actress' partner. Remaining 'not in the know', even for a moment, may stir curiosity, which could of course be healthy, but for my patient it is so much suffused with hostility and spoiling that it becomes perverse, sexualised and prurient. It means our minds cannot work separately and his relate to

171

mine comfortably and he use his interest and curiosity constructively and creatively. Thus communication between us must become barren, there can be no creative thought only a kind of paralysis. And there are other dangers about being 'in the know' connected with being understood. There are times when I interpret something and Mr A falls silent, as if pulling away from me. Sometimes it is then possible to see that my understanding has become too close, felt by him as too physical and in that sense seductive, so in order to avoid being engulfed and trapped he withdraws into his own thinking, usually intellectualisations.

I have tried to show the kind of anxieties that underlie Mr A's personality organisation and something of the defences that he uses to maintain his precarious balance. I want, before ending, to bring a dream which I think illustrates this balance rather clearly.

> In the dream there was a solid iron or steel framework, it looked like a picture frame but must have had seats as he had the habit of using it to travel on the underground train lines. Then he thought why not try it on the main railway lines? So he went to South London which seemed to be in the country (he lives in North London). But then he was in a panic, how to get back, how to manage the main line points etc. how to get onto the tube line again? He was somewhere unknown to him, but he got out and talked to a man who invited him to his lodgings for a meal. He went with this man but quickly got the impression that the latter was mentally ill, out of touch with reality and constantly getting stuck in the same sentence. The man went out of the room and my patient took the opportunity to try to go downstairs and escape, but he met the man coming up. He let go of the metal frame which fell, he caught it as it was about to hit the man, but he was not quite in time and it banged his shin.

He woke convinced that his own shin was hurt. In his associations which I cannot give in detail, he spoke about an apparently mentally ill old man, whom he often meets in the street near his office – but the man in the dream was his own age.

I think that my patient here shows unconscious insight into his own dilemma. He knows, unconsciously, that he is living in a rigid steel framework, in his obsessional defensive world, and that he travels through life with it, underground, unobserved. He feels he wants to come out into the main stream of life, the main life of relating – but if he goes too far, and the analysis might take him too far – how will he get back to his familiar ground, his familiar ways? He shows us the dangers and the dilemma – breakdown, mental illness. If he gets out of his perverse obsessional state he fears having to face the mentally ill man, the ill part of himself and how out of touch with reality and how stuck in a repetitive mode he is. But he cannot escape what he sees, he tries to but the man comes back, the illness has to be faced. If he holds onto the metal frame he believes it gives safety, but he knows it damages him, if he lets go it damages the man in the dream, his own shin as it emerges as he wakes.

There is another warning here, I think, that unless I as his analyst, can get through his rigid control, to the mentally ill part, that is through the obsessional and perverse aspects, I shall be stuck for ever, analysing on the same rigid lines and the analysis will be just the frame that supports him, a crutch that must be there for ever.

The dream then exemplifies some of the dangers that beset this patient, particularly the danger and the importance of facing his own mentally ill state, which for moments we can make contact with as I tried to illustrate in the material earlier. Really facing this means holding onto insight into himself, which is very difficult to achieve. He will see something for a moment but then it gets lost, intellectualised, turned into dry words instead of leading to real seeing – to vision. If he is to join the main stream of life, relating, it will mean connecting up with real people, not just objects he can use in his own way to carry projected aspects of himself, or objects that he can get into and from whom he can take over what he needs to feed his superiority and omnipotence.

In this paper I start from a very simple example of the sexualisation of thinking and of the transference and describe how it is essentially anti-sexuality and anti-creativity. I discuss how sexualisation, like perversion, of which it is one aspect cannot be considered in isolation but how it is part of a whole personality organisation which I try to describe using material from a second and more obviously disturbed case. I describe how this patient Mr A cannot relate to an object which is separate and at a distance from him, objects can only be related to in a superficial or excited, sexualised manner, symbolised by the masturbatory movement of finger to finger. Penetration is equated with being invaded and taken over and leads to panic and fear of a confusional state or breakdown. But preventing it leads to neutering and paralysis. The result is that there can be no genuine sexuality, no intercourse, only perverse sexuality. In the analysis the analyst's mind and thoughts are not allowed to feed or connect up with the patient's and nourish or produce new generations of thought, vision in this way is prevented and new ideas, the people, perish.

Reason and Passion

Acknowledgement

An earlier version of this chapter was written for a symposium on 'From Sexualisation to Erotic Desire' held at Columbia University, New York in 1994.

References

Freud, S. (1910) 'The Psycho-Analytic View of Psychogenic Disturbance of Vision', *S.E.* 11, 209-18.
—— (1915) 'Observations on Transference Love', *S.E.* 12, 157-71.
Segal, H. (1981) *Delusion and Artistic Creativity*, Free Association Books and Maresfield Library.
—— (1991) *Dream, Phantasy and Art*. London: Tavistock/Routledge.

Acknowledgements

The following kindly gave permission to use previously published material: Institute of Psycho-Analysis, The International Universities Press and Jason Aronson.

O'Shaugnessy, E. (1992) 'Enclaves and excursions', *International Journal of Psycho-Analysis* 73: 603-61, © Institute of Psycho-Analysis.

Sohn, L. (1995) 'Unprovoked assaults-making sense of apparently random violence', *International Journal of Psycho-Analysis* 5 76:565-575, © Institute of Psycho-Analysis.

Riesenberg Malcolm, R. (1980) 'Expiation as a defence', *International Journal of Psychoanalytic Psychotherapy*, 8:549-570, © Jason Aronson.

Anderson, R. (1997) 'Putting the Boot in: violent defences against depressive anxiety' in Schafer, R. ed., *The Contemporary Kleinians of London*. Madison: International Universities Press, © International Universities Press.

'Blocked Introjection/Blocked Incorporation' Schafer, R. (1997) in *The Contemporary Kleinians of London*. Madison: International Universities Press, © International Universities Press.

Select Bibliography of the Work of Hanna Segal

Books

1964   *Introduction to the Work of Melanie Klein*. London: Hogarth Press.
1979   *Klein*. London: Fontana.
1981   *The Work of Hanna Segal*. New York: Jason Aronson, Repr. (1986). London: Free Association Books and Maresfield Library.
1991   *Dream, Phantasy and Art*. London: Routledge.
1997   *Psychoanalysis, Literature and War*. London: Routledge.

Chapters in Books

1989   'Political Thinking : Psychoanalytic Perspectives' in Basnett, L. and Leigh, I. eds, *Political Thinking*. London: Pluto Press.
1990   'Psychoanalysis and Freedom of Thought' in Sandler, J. ed., *Dimensions of Psychoanalysis*. Madison: International Universities Press.
1991   'The Theory of Narcissism in the Work of Freud and Klein' with Bell, D. in Sandler, J., Person, E.S. and Fonagy, P. eds, *Freud's 'On Narcissism: An Introduction'*. London: Yale.
1992   'Acting on Phantasy and Acting on Desire' in Hopkins, J. and Savile, A. eds, *Psychoanalysis, Mind and Art: Perspectives on Richard Wollheim*. Oxford: Blackwell.
1993   'Countertransference' in Alexandris, A. and Vaslamatzis, G. eds, *Countertransference: Theory, Technique, Teaching*. London: Karnac.
1994   'Paranoid Anxiety and Paranoia' in Oldham, J.M. and Bone, S. eds, *Paranoia: New Psychoanalytic Perspectives*. Madison: International Universities Press.
1995   'Hiroshima, the Gulf War and after' in Elliot, A. and Frosh, S. eds, *Psychoanalysis in Contexts: Paths between Theory and Modern Culture*. London: Routledge.
1997   'Manic Reparation' in Schafer, R. ed., *The Contemporary Kleinians of London*. Madison: International Universities Press.

Select Bibliography of the Work of Hanna Segal

Articles

1950 'Some aspects of the analysis of a schizophrenic', *International Journal of Psycho-Analysis*, 31: 268-278.

1951 Review of Winnicott, D., *The Ordinary Devoted Mother and her Baby: Nine Broadcast Talks* in: *International Journal of Psycho-Analysis*, 32: 327-328.

1952 'A psychoanalytical approach to aesthetics', *International Journal of Psycho-Analysis*, 33: 96-297.

1953 'A necrophilic phantasy', *International Journal of Psycho-Analysis*, 34: 98-101.

1954 'A note on schizoid mechanisms underlying phobia formation', *International Journal of Psycho-Analysis*, 35: 238-241.

1956 'Depression in the schizophrenic', *International Journal of Psycho-Analysis*, 37: 339-343.

1957 'Notes on symbol formation', *International Journal of Psycho-Analysis*, 38: 391-397.

1958 'Fear of death: notes on the analysis of an old man', *International Journal of Psycho-Analysis*, 39 178-181.

1962 'The curative factors in psychoanalysis', *International Journal of Psycho-Analysis*, 43:212-217.

1964 'Symposium on phantasy', *International Journal of Psycho-Analysis*,45: 191-194.

1972 'A delusional system as a defence against the re-emergence of a catastrophic situation', *International Journal of Psycho-Analysis*, 53:393-402.

1972 'Role of child analysis in the general psychoanalytic training', *International Journal of Psycho-Analysis*, 53: 157-161.

1974 'Delusion and artistic creativity: *The Spire* by W. Golding', *International Review of Psychoanalysis*, 1: 135-141.

1977 'Psychoanalytic dialogue; Kleinian theory today', *Journal of the American Psychoanalytical. Association*, 25: 363-370.

1978 'On symbolism', *International Journal of Psycho-Analysis*, 59: 315-320.

1981 'Interpretation and primitive psychic processes: a Kleinian view' with Britton, R., *Psychoanalytical Inquiry*, 1: 267-268.

1982 'Early infantile development as reflected in the psychoanalytic process: steps in integration', *International Journal of Psycho-Analysis*, 63: 15-22.

1983 'Clinical implications of Melanie Klein's work: emergence from narcissism', *International Journal of Psycho-Analysis*, 64: 269-276.

1984 'Joseph Conrad and the mid-life crisis', *International Review of Psychoanalysis*, 11: 3-10.

1987 'Silence is the real crime', *International Review of Psychoanalysis*, 14: 3-12.

1988 'Sweating it out', *Psychoanalytical Study of Children*, 43: 167-178.

1990 'Some comments on the Alexander technique', *Psychoanalytical Inquiry*, 10: 409-414.
1990 'How theory shapes technique: a Kleinian view', with Roth. P, *Psychoanalytical Inquiry*, 10: 541-549.
1990 'El complex d'Edip avui', *Revista catalana de psiconalasi*, 7(2) : 273-280.
1991 'Psychoanalyse et therapeutique', *Revue française de psychoanalyse*, 2: 366-376.
1992 'The achievement of ambivalence', *Common Knowledge*, 1: 92-104.
1993 On the clinical usefulness of the concept of the death instinct', *International Journal of Psycho-Analysis*, 74: 55-62.
1993 'A transferencia na psicanalise da crianca' with O'Shaugnessy, E., *Revista brasiliera de psicanalise*, 27: 141-158.
1994 'Salman Rushdie and the sea of stories', *International Journal of Psycho-Analysis*, 75: 611-618.
1994 'Phantasy and reality', *International Journal of Psycho-Analysis*, 75: 359-401.

TAVISTOCK CLINIC SERIES

Also available:

MULTIPLE VOICES
Narrative in Systemic Family Therapy
Edited by Renos Papadopoulos and John Byng-Hall

This book offers a comprehensive overview of issues related to narrative which appear in a family therapy setting. Originally embarking on a joint project to share clinical experience, members of the Family Systems Group at the Tavistock Clinic discovered that what was common in their work was their emphasis on narrative. This discovery led, in time, to the development of a shared discourse about their diverse approaches to narrative which are carefully reflected in the contributions in this volume. Part One sets out the context of narrative with contributions on bilingualism and the family's experience of therapy, ending with a thought-provoking critique of narrative. Part Two concentrates on applications of these ideas, providing analysis of multiple narratives in illness and loss, gender and language, neonatal care, adoption, divorce and refugee families.

Renos Papadopoulos is a Consultant Clinical Psychologist at the Tavistock Clinic and Professor of Analytical Psychology at the University of Essex. **John Byng-Hall** is a Consultant Child and Family Psychiatrist at the Tavistock Clinic and is a Past Chair of the Institute of Family Therapy in London.

The editors and all contributors are systemic family psychotherapists, coming from a variety of professional backgrounds and work at the Child and Family Therapy Department at the Tavistock Clinic as clinicians and trainers. All belong to research teams within the Family Systems Group at the Tavistock Clinic involved on a long-term basis with research into narrative in family psychotherapy.

ISBN: 0-7156-2777-5   Published: September 1997   £12.95

Duckworth Publishers
48 Hoxton Square, London N1 6PB
Tel: 0171 729 5986

179

PSYCHOTIC STATES IN CHILDREN

Edited by Margaret Rustin, Maria Rhode,
Alex Dubinsky and Hélène Dubinsky

There is something extremely unsettling about the disturbed behaviour of sexually abused and severely troubled children. In spite of a sometimes exasperating measure of perversion and destructive wilfulness, these children manage to communicate a clear plea for help – a plea which deeply affects those in their immediate surroundings who find themselves struggling to make sense of these contradictory messages. This book describes significant new developments in the understanding and psychotherapeutic treatment of children and adolescents suffering from psychotic levels of disturbance.

Each chapter contains a clinical description of a child emerging from a psychotic state, creating a useful collection of case histories. Part One concerns sexually abused children, Part Two discusses children with severe developmental delay, and Part Three describes the treatment of children whose difficulties have both internal and external roots. Each Part is followed by an authoritative critical commentary. A glossary of terms used is included at the end of the book.

Margaret Rustin and **Maria Rhode** are Consultant Child Psychotherapists in the Child and Family Department at the Tavistock Clinic. **Hélène Dubinsky** is a Consultant Child Psychotherapist in the Adolescent Department at the Tavistock Clinic. **Alex Dubinsky** is a Child Psychotherapist and is a tutor at the Tavistock Clinic.

ISBN: 0-7156-2775-9   Published: September 1997   £12.95

INTERNAL LANDSCAPES AND FOREIGN BODIES
Eating Disorders and other Pathologies
By Gianna Williams

Klein's model of projective and introjective processes and Bion's model of the relationship between container and contained have become increasingly significant in much clinical work. In a highly imaginative development of these models of thought, the distinguished clinician Gianna Williams, one of the leading figures in the field, elucidates the psychodynamics of these processes in the context of impairment of dependent relationships and eating disorders in both men and women. This is a timely and brilliant account of an area of psychopathology that is rapidly growing in significance.

Gianna Williams is a Consultant Child and Adolescent Psychotherapist in the Adolescent Department at the Tavistock Clinic and Professor with tenure at Pisa University, Italy. She is also founder of the Eating Disorder Workshop set up in 1987 and has lectured widely and influentially on these themes in Europe and Latin America.

ISBN: 0-7156-2781-3   Published: November 1997   £12.95

Available from spring 1998:

UNDERSTANDING TRAUMA
A Psychoanalytical Approach
Edited by Caroline Garland

Major disasters draw attention forcibly to their effects on the survivor. Less visible are the trauma and after-effects of non-public events. Understanding the nature of this kind of breakdown is essential if treatment is to be effective and durable. This book describes, through an interweaving of theory and practice, work ranging from a short series of therapeutic consultations to full analysis.

Caroline Garland is a Consultant Clinical Psychoanalyst and Psychologist and founder of the Unit for the Study of Trauma and its Aftermath in the Adult Department of the Tavistock Clinic.

ISBN: 0-7156-2776-7   £14.95

DEVELOPMENT OF THE PERSONALITY
Psychoanalysis and the Growth of the Mind
By Margot Waddell

Following the major developmental phases from infancy to old age, the author lucidly explores those vital aspects of experience which promote mental and emotional growth and those which impede it. The book traces the interplay between factors, internal and external, which contribute to a person's character strength and sense of identity. The book offers a detailed and accessible introduction to contemporary psychoanalytic thought while at the same time its breadth will engage readers from an academic context, the professional practitioner and the concerned parent. In bringing together a wide range of clinical, non-clinical and literary examples it provides a personal and vivid perspective on the relationship between psychodynamic theory and the nature of human development.

Margot Waddell is a Psycho-Analyst and Consultant Child Psychotherapist in the Adolescent Department at the Tavistock Clinic.

ISBN: 0-7156-2823-2   £14.95

FACING IT OUT
Disruptive Adolescents From a Clinical Perspective
Edited by Robin Anderson and Anna Dartington

With the exception of infancy, adolescence is the most radical of all developmental periods. The Adolescent Department in its long history has been engaging with young people and their families when the strains prove too great. In this book, staff of the Department describe a range of disturbances from adjustment crises to anorexia nervosa and psychosis.

Robin Anderson is a Consultant Child and Adolescent Psychiatrist and Chairman of the Adolescent Department as well as a Training Analyst in child and adult analysis at the British Psycho-Analytical Society.

Anna Dartington is a Psychoanalytic Psychotherapist and Chair of two Tavistock Clinical Services, The Young People's Counselling Service and the Psychoanalytic Family Workshop.

ISBN: 0-7156-2794-5   £14.95